TABLE OF CONTENTS

MELANCHOLIA

For Chris, Ben, and Paul

Introduction

Melancholia is a series of essays about clinical depression. It arose from a great loneliness, and the far off yet singular belief that maybe someday my experiences could help someone else.

I have been a depressive as far back as I can remember; to the point at which the experiences generated are a large part of who I am. It wasn't until my early thirties and having kids that it got so bad I had to seek help. I remember leaning against the green and white tiles of the kitchen counter, the late afternoon sun streaming through the window illuminating the grease spots on the stove of our first tiny adobe house. I hid it fairly well but a full blown psychological break was imminent.

I hadn't slept for days, couldn't carry out the most routine functions or care about any topic of conversation. I wept at the slightest prompting and sometimes for no reason at all. The world was grey and drained of color. I couldn't remember what joy was.

That moment is as acute in my memory as the moment before impact in a car crash. It was like the instant when time slows down to an absolute crawl and you know with utter certainty not just that you're going to hit, but that it's going to be bad. My grasp on reality in that instant, as the result of prolonged despair and the whopping amount of fear that comes with motherhood, was slipping like wheels on an oil slick right out from under me.

I later discovered I was in the throes of a major depression. I couldn't recognize it; didn't even know there was such a thing. You see, I was just myself only more so, sort of like double pneumonia is just a head cold only more so, and couldn't perceive how drastically things had gone wrong. I realize now that being seriously depressed was ultimately totally consistent my definition of self.

So I had to redefine myself. Not reinvent. It's an important difference. Reinvention implies a degree of artifice. Redefinition is about coming at who you are from a new angle.

Along the way I took notes.

When I was in the worst of it: when the Selective Serotonin Re-uptake Inhibitors weren't working; when crackpot psychologists were expounding theories I knew weren't true, when acupuncturists were sticking pins in me, I wrote it all down. When I was ill. When I was feeling better. When I had reached the surrealistic wall that *is* HMOs and mental illness, I wrote. Since reading William James in college, I have always liked the essay form. So I wrote essays.

I am not a psychologist or an MD. I'm an ex-Roman Catholic with a degree in philosophy with a further emphasis in classics. Some of these essays have been revised, mostly to remove tirades at the gods, maudlin speculation, and swear words though some persist. I am, at core, a potty mouth and apologize to more sensitive souls in advance.

Peace, Catherine O'Sullivan

July, 2005

Hazards and Headshrinkers

We all need someone we can bleed on. Mick Jagger was right.

But it's not as easy as you might think. There are all kinds of people out there able to get through degree programs and hang out shingles calling themselves *psychologists*. The problem with some of them however, is that they are just individuals trying to figure out the roots of their own pain, with varying degrees of success. They won't admit this, to themselves or anyone else. But those on the low end of the success curve can do a lot of damage. In short, you can't learn to become sane from someone who's nuttier than you are.

Anyone who's got their own soul sealed off is incapable of piercing yours.

There are many ways to tell you're mired in a major depression. Some people can't get out of bed. Some people eat too much, drink too much booze and do drugs. Some get severe insomnia. The last happened to me and I went to my HMO doctor. He proceeded to completely miss the depression and wrote me a prescription for sleeping pills. I got addicted to the sleeping pills, quit after a few weeks and went through withdrawals, only to find that I was still depressed, but more so than ever.

I was so angry with the "medical establishment," that I went to a psychologist trained in acupuncture. One of my touchier, feelier, friends had been at me for months waving herbs under my nose, pushing at so-called pressure points and telling me my chakras were blocked. Hell, as far as I could tell, my whole life was blocked. I was positively paralyzed by melancholy, perched upon that razor's edge that only the truly down and borderline psychotic can know.

Still I was skeptical, especially when I saw all those needles, but figured hey, I'm already in pain, what's a little more?

I lay down on the table and a stooped, middle-aged man who looked like Zero Mostel came in, chatting up a storm about how I'd made the right decision, about how the medical establishment had become so corrupted by the insurance industry and drug companies there was no reasoning with it. Why, the patient was at the very bottom of the list of their concerns, as far as he could tell. He fiddled about the room, gathering his tools, humming "The Girl from Ipanema." Then he approached twiddling a fistful of needles. They were about a quarter of the thickness of the average straight pin. He proceeded to stick the whole bunch of them in me: a few in the ears, more in the legs, an unknown number in the arms.

He told me to lay there awhile, to just relax in order for the treatment to work. Fine, I said, no problem. At least with all those pins sticking in me, I was no longer preoccupied with hiding the fact that as a result of drug addiction, lack of sleep, appetite, and that overall spiky aspect the world takes on when all the trappings of rest and good cheer have dropped off, I was as close to losing it as I'd ever been.

And just as I'd finished counting the first hundred holes in the ceiling tiles, the man started telling me about his own depression.

It seemed Herr Acupuncturist's dear mother was killed in a traffic accident. Oh, he went into all the gory details: what limbs came off—right arm and left foot, or visa versa, the alcohol content of the guy's blood who caused it, the close bond he had with dear old Mum (which he was convinced he'd never again attain with anyone, not in this life anyway.) He described the unfeeling paramedics, the lackadaisical emergency room staff, the weather, the humidity, the particulate matter contained in the air of the city that day.

And there I was, pinned to the table like a bug, a captive audience.

All this treatment got me was a hundred fifty dollars poorer, maybe a little more awareness of the danger at the intersection of the Campbell and Twelfth Avenues, and dozens of holes in my hide.

Picture St. Sebastian, only female and the holes are smaller; but the eyes cast heavenwards in exactly the same way.

Then there was the guy with the biofeedback machines. Ph.D., tall man, very authoritative, yet gentle in his demeanor.

This is the point at which I should have turned around and walked out the door—the point at which I became aware enough of the man's physicality to put words to it. Not that I was attracted him, it was the way he carried himself—like my father—and he had that wounded, desperate look in his eyes. I figured him for a Vietnam vet long before he ever told me he was. He was the right age and clearly had that military stiffness thing going. As a result, *I felt for him*. Give me a damaged guy and I am powerless, like Superman around kryptonite.

I don't want to think about how powerless I was: about fifteen hundred dollars powerless, doled out in hundred dollar increments over a period of months.

I'd come in weeping, he'd hook me to a machine, tell me to generate alpha brain waves. I'm not bragging but I'm from Southern California, so I can do the touchy-feely pseudoscientific shit standing on my head. It's like someone from a farm in Indiana knowing how to drive a tractor. So I'd generate the damn brainwaves and when he asked if I was feeling better, I'd say *yes*. I didn't want to disappoint the poor guy, who to be honest, looked more depressed than I did.

The next week I'd come back, and we'd do the same thing. About five hundred dollars along, I finally admitted to Dr Victnam that the machine wasn't working. That's when he started in on the nutritional supplements.

In those days I still wanted to embrace a mechanistic view of human beings simply because I knew I was broken, and a machine can be fixed. So I took the calcium, the St. John's Wort, the melatonin, the selenium, the tryptophane precursor, whatever that was. I abstained from demon caffeine, red meat, alcohol. I exercised every day, but I do that anyway.

And at the next appointment I'd be back, weeping. He'd ask me if I was doing any better and even though I wanted to scream, "Do I look like I'm doing any fucking better?" I'd say, "ah, maybe."

Then one day he told me of the wonders of a machine I could rent from him (for only a hundred dollars a month), which would surely do the trick. You clip it on your earlobes and it generates tiny electrical impulses that penetrate your brain and straighten things out. I said, "Well, if there is such a device, how come I've never heard of it?" (*n.b.*: clinical depression lowers your IQ about fifty points.). He said it was widely used in Russia, but suppressed in the United States due to a conspiracy involving the government and the big pharmaceutical companies. (Another *n.b.*: These alternative medicine guys need to come up with something besides the "it's widely used in Russia," line. It worked well-enough when Russia was a socialist utopia, handing out wondrous medical devices like day-old bread, but now? The average Russian doesn't look so happy to me, and I don't picture him being able to afford one of these gizmos. Even if he could, he'd probably get an iPod instead. I would.

Two hundred dollars later, I told him, "this thing doesn't work."

That was the beginning of the end for me and Dr Vietnam. I was in a session, playing with a Rubic's cube while he told me of a miracle "nutritional supplement" called GHB (put "date rape drug" into any computer search engine and it will find it in about a half a second). I experienced a barely controllable urge to throw the aforementioned cube at the good doctor as hard as I could.

The story does have a happy ending. I emigrated to Russia, where

I have all these incredible medical devices at my disposal every day.

Actually, I found a nurse practitioner who got me on some meds that actually worked and helped me find a competent psychologist. The psychologist told me that yes, I could get outside all this pain but it's going to be hard work. I had no idea at the time, but this was the equivalent of a Pole in 1939 telling his neighbor he figured there might be a war coming.

Anti-Depressants: What They Do

Anti-depressants seem to be everywhere these days. Is this because they're being over-prescribed? Undoubtedly; and there are probably many people on them who would be better off with psychotherapy or lesser treatments. But I think a more significant factor is the advent of SSRI's or Selective Serotonin Re-uptake Inhibitors. This new generation of drugs simply does not have the side effects of the old ones, which were so numerous and severe that almost no one would take them. Once upon a time, depressed persons had to be committed to mental institutions to get treatment; or be otherwise so disabled their loved ones didn't know what to do with them.

It's not a bad thing that help is more readily available now. Whether taking anti-depressant medication is right or wrong, I'm not going to get into. In the end it's a personal decision as are most things. But it bothers me that most of the patter about such medications, even that coming from over-worked and harried doctors, comes from the pharmaceutical companies that manufacture them. Pharmaceutical representatives not only stock physicians' pantries, but take entire medical office staffs to lunch regularly, thereby coercing them to use an increasing amount of their products. These guys make kids from the 'hood look like rank amateurs when it comes to pushing drugs; and most MD's know next to nothing about mental illness. This makes for a dangerous combination.

So herein are the anti-depressants I've had experience with. This list is not meant to be either comprehensive or complete.

Prozac is by far the most common and well known of the new breed of anti-depressants, and in my opinion a very good one. However, it doesn't work for everybody and many complain it puts the kibosh on their sex drive. This is obviously a depressing development (or non-development as the case may be), and I wouldn't blame anyone for finding it unacceptable in the long run. If it works otherwise, sometimes doctors mix a little Welbutrin with it. This worked extremely well for me, and on second thought too well. I think it had me propositioning every moderately attractive sentient being with whom I came into contact. I read an article by a woman who claims with Welbutrin added to her SSRI, caused her to experience a two hour orgasms at the shopping mall. She said it only happened once and that afterwards, her sex drive returned to "a normal if somewhat heightened state." Brain chemistry is delicate and a still poorly understood thing. So with any medication it's important to pay close attention to your real reactions, and not to what other people tell you they're supposed to be.

The drawback with Welbutrin comes into play if you're a drinker. If you mix Welbutrin with alcohol, it can cause seizures. This has been well documented. Interestingly enough however, this need not be a problem since the drug also lessens your cravings for drugs including nicotine and alcohol. Welbutrin, called Zyban in stop-smoking ads, is one of the medications given to people detox. For some individuals it also lessens the cravings for unnecessary food thereby helping them lose weight. I lost interest in food altogether, which was no fun. I couldn't stay on it as a result.

The only tricyclic I've tried was Trazedone, which didn't work. Tricyclic anti-depressants were the generation before SSRI's, and before that it was MAO inhibitors. Contrary to popular belief, MAO inhibitors have nothing to do with Chinese communism in the sixties. Most doctors don't prescribe them anymore because it's not just alcohol with which they combine badly, though they do, But many foods and beverages in combination with MAO's, cause serious illness. Both MAO inhibitors and tricyclic anti-depressants cause dry mouth and often, weight gain. The latter is enough to send most women spiraling into moderate depression all by itself.

There's another problem with tricyclics that bears mentioning. They are great for committing suicide, beating valium and Co-Tylenol by miles. If you wind up in an emergency room with a belly full of tricyclics, there is very little the doctors can do. It seems a little odd, giving a seriously depressed person something so good for ending it all, and a big drawback if they don't work and you've got three quarters of a bottle hanging around the house. Of course, one could say the same thing about Lysol. People who genuinely want to do themselves in usually find a way.

Before we leave Prozac completely behind, here's a personal

anecdote. I'd been on Prozac for about seven years when it stopped working. It was a very gradual thing, either physiologically or psychologically, I'm not sure which. It could be that it was an all of the sudden thing, and I just wasn't aware of it for a year or so because I didn't want to believe it. I told myself that sitting at the kitchen table at two in the morning wishing for oblivion, wondering how in the hell I could ever get out from underneath all this pain, was a transient thing. It's important to understand that for me, finding Prozac was like finding Jesus, only it worked.

So by the time I did make it to the shrink, I was pretty much a wrecked shell of a human being, lost, confused, and exhausted. The shrink told me they had recently discovered a phenomenon called 'Prozac poop-out,' (isn't that *cute!*), and that for some reason not understood by medical science, **sometimes it just quits on people.** He thought he could fix the problem by doubling my daily dose.

After about a week on the increased dosage I didn't feel any better, but knew I had to give it time. You have to give the older SSRI's at least six weeks and I was familiar enough with the drill to just hunker down and wait. Then one night after dinner, I snapped the leashes on my dogs and headed out the door to take them for a walk. Damned if the minute I closed the front door behind me, a Stealth Bomber didn't come out of nowhere, buzz me from about 200 feet and disappear behind my house. I flattened myself on the ground like a rabbit beneath the shadow of a hawk.

My dogs looked at me like I had lost my damn mind, which I had.

It seems that too much Prozac can cause hallucinations. They don't tell you that going in, but when I mentioned it to the shrink who prescribed it he said, "ah yes, that is a possible side effect." Side effect, side effect! I can handle a hallucination or two—I grew up in the 70's—but I can't very well go through life thinking large military aircraft are coming out of nowhere now can I? Side effect my Aunt Fanny. I mean, in the best case it's embarrassing, in the worst case I could have broken my front teeth on the cement.

A word about shrinks, actually three words: I hate them. Not psychologists, although eighty percent of them are nuts right out of the chute and any reasonable person should probably have nothing to do with them, but *psychiatrists*. In these HMO days they are mostly MD's who took a seminar or two on psychiatry. Not only do they not care about you, they are generally so wedded to a completely mechanistic view of human beings, including themselves, that they are incapable of empathy with anyone. In fact, they have nothing but disdain for you, the nut-case, because they have their own heads sealed up so tightly they've convinced themselves they're immune to whatever psychosis or neurosis you're presenting. *You therefore scare the shit out of them.*

Mine actually got mad at me because the stuff he tried wasn't working. His attitude was "you dumb hysteric, don't you know this stuff works?!" He tried Serzone. Nothing. Paxil made me so constipated I wished for the depression back. Remeron made me gain ten pounds and unable to think about anything but food and sex.

Finally I got connected with a nurse practitioner trained in psychiatry. She talked to me for a half an hour, pinpointed the problems, gave me the right prescriptions. In my experience, such people are usually in the so-called "helping" professions because they genuinely want to help. I've argued with people over this but to my way of thinking, an ounce of genuine empathy is worth more than a memorized Physicians Desk Reference any day.

Sometimes you have to try several things before you know what's right for you, and chances are, whatever you take, there will be side effects. I make a distinction between acceptable and unacceptable side effects. Right now I'm on Zoloft, which does diminish my sex drive a little, *diminish* being the operative word. I still enjoy sex, it just takes a little longer to get going. To me, this is an acceptable side effect. Maybe for a thin person who doesn't mind gaining a few pounds, Remeron would be just fine. The important point is that **since fifteen percent of severely depressed people commit suicide,** some side effects are probably a reasonable trade off.

Whoever is treating you, at the very least make sure he or she is of moderate intelligence and open to discussion. For example, if you tell them you're so depressed your sex drive is gone and this really upsets you, and they write a script for Prozac, the medication that seems to effect patients sex drive the most, they are not listening. If you're athletic or vain, both of which I am, and the idea of being fat is abhorrent to you and they prescribe an anti-depressant like Remeron—where weight is a known and common side effect—again they aren't hearing you. Every shrink and MD, even if it's your gynecologist writing out the prescription, has a preferred method of treatment based on averages of his or her experience. Whoever you are, **you are not average**.

If they don't believe you, you might try humping over, making a horrible face and, like the Elephant Man, screaming—I am a human being! It worked for me and chances are, you'll get what you need, if for no other reason than to stop you from coming back in a hurry.

Corkscrewed Neurons

So the other day, I'm reading the New Yorker magazine and there's an article about depression. Said article warned me I might be ruining my brain with Selective Serotonin Re-uptake Inhibitors.

I am not greedy. When I hit thirty-three, I realized I'd lived longer than both Jesus Christ and Alexander the Great. At forty, I'd passed John Lennon. At forty-five I have beaten John Kennedy by two years (what do I win?) If you step back from human history and give it a good hard stare you'll find that statistically, most people get twenty or thirty years if they're lucky. Longevity is a comparatively modern invention. I figure that's why seventeen, eighteen year-old guys think about sex all the time. During the millions years of pre-agricultural human evolution, males almost never lasted longer than that, and had to spread their genes before getting trampled by mastodons or rogue prehistoric yaks. Women? Before modern obstetrics, childbirth and its complications generally got them.

The point is, thirty-five or forty thousand years ago, finding anybody over thirty was tough. But don't feel bad because for animals it's worse. My cat will probably get twelve, fifteen years unless he gets eaten by a coyote. The coyote, whether he eats my cat or not, will probably get considerably less. If I live long enough to get my kids raised, which statistically I probably will, I'll feel pretty lucky. If I make it to seventy or eighty, which again I expect to, that'll be fine. But—and this is a big but—I want to do it with my mental faculties intact. I mean let's face it, you can spend your whole life being brilliant but spend a couple of years at the end telling everyone you meet about the death rays coming from your aluminum cookware or the aliens trying to take over your brain, and that's all they'll remember.

"Oh, those last couple of years were tough," they'll say. "She ever start babbling about the aluminum thing and the aliens when you were around? Yeah, sad wasn't it." That's it, that's all you'll get. Think about Stephen Hawking—a truly brilliant theoretical astrophysicist and if you mention his name to someone they'll generally say something along the lines of, "Oh, yeah, isn't he that smart guy in the wheelchair?" Not one person will be able to tell you what he works on, most won't even know what kind of scientist he is. They just know he's crippled and talks through a computer that buzzes.

Of course this New Yorker article did not say definitively that SSRI's are ruining my brain. What it said is that nobody knows what the long term effects of them are because they haven't been around long enough to be thoroughly studied. It said that if you give a rat one hundred times the average recommended dose of Prozac for four days then dissect its brain, "the neurons exhibit corkscrew like profiles."

Now obviously no one takes a hundred times the prescribed dose of Prozac, but then again, they do take it longer than four days. When I first started taking it, an MD told me it wasn't dangerous at all, that even if I tried to kill myself by taking a whole bottle of the stuff it wouldn't do a thing. Well excuse me, but I don't think neurons with "corkscrew-like profiles" is nothing.

Here's a cute story, and it isn't a non-sequitur so bear with me. My maternal grandmother, an otherwise gentile woman, used to snore like a truck driver at the end of three day drunk. It was astounding. I remember thinking the first time I spent the night at her house, I should sleep with the covers over my head so that when the ceiling started coming down I wouldn't breathe the dust. Years later when she was old, tied to her chair in the nursing home with no idea who I was, I learned that she'd been taking barbiturates since the nineteen fifties "for a stomach ailment." Aha, no wonder Grandma used to get so bombed off a couple of sherries before dinner. It's a miracle she could sit up through the entire meal.

Of course, I now I know why she took those downers: Grandma couldn't sleep (insomnia is one of several symptoms of depression), just like her mother—who wrote long letters detailing the misery of her chronic insomnia—just like my mother who blamed it on me for staying out too late. Some doctor, well meaning I imagine, got Grandma junked out on downers and she never got off them. I'm sure he told her they were perfectly safe and not to worry.

I don't know much about my own mother's history of drug use but I do remember that just about everybody else's mom back in the late sixties and early seventies had a prescription for Valium. Only they called it "tranquilizers." *Tranquil,* isn't that a nice word? I'd love to be tranquil, sitting on the forest floor, dappled sunlight all round, butterflies dancing in the warm spring breeze, my biggest concern whether or not to turn the page of some Walt Whitman poem that goes on for eight hundred pages. Ah, *tranquil.* Watch a few old movies and every time a woman has a crisis, kindly yet authoritative Doctor Black-bag is always at her bedside administering "tranquilizers" and patting her hand.

Lemme tell you, some of those moms back in the old days were damn tranquil. Plenty of them were unconscious. Of course the selling point for benzodiazepines, Valium and the like, was that *though they might be habit-forming they weren't addictive.* Whatever that means.

There are no people on earth with the kind of two dimensional mindsets of Americans. Black and white, the good guys and the bad, either/or. Thinking this way gives us time for watching TV, buying electronics and big cars. Communism as an economic system was a seventy year experiment that seemed to have ended badly for many people. But, that doesn't mean that unrestrained capitalism is good. Economic systems have no morality and capitalism is no exception. Its single imperative is to make as much money as possible for the *people with the capital.* And *"capital"* don't mean a few thousand bucks. It means millions, generally residing in the hands of individuals who would sell their own grandmothers to the Visalia chapter of the Hell's Angels for the inside track on hot new pharmaceutical stock.

They would have you think otherwise, "what, who us? Nah, we're nice guys who wear expensive suits and golf"; basically they think of you and I not so much as fellow human beings but as marks; and if you don't believe it then you are the very person PT Barnum was talking about. Only these days there's one born every thirty seconds.

These are the very people, by the way, for whom in the event of some unanticipated mental scramble, affording high-priced psychiatrists with balanced views and information is not a problem. You and I on the other hand get over-worked, fast-food care givers down to the local HMO and treatments the biggest selling point of which is efficacy and low-cost. If down the road Prozac becomes the Dalcon Shield of the twenty first century all we'll get is a big fat *WHOOPS!*

I remember a few years ago, I was about thirty-five. (Funny how *a few* can become, ten.) Anyway, I had been on Prozac for a few months and I slept in. I woke up feeling a little weird, the way you do when you normally get up at six but find yourself still abed at eight. Suddenly I got this funny sort-of shaking feeling in my head. It didn't hurt, but I didn't like it. It lasted maybe five, seven seconds. When I got up and tried to read I couldn't. The lines on the page looked disjointed, cracked down the middle. Needless to say it scared me.

Now it could have been any number of things. I've lived an active life and been knocked in the head more times than I can remember, but at the time I wondered if it was the Prozac so I called the nurse at my HMO and asked her. She read from her handout—I could hear her lips moving—and told me that no, it was not possible, that if I'd had some kind of *cerebral event*, it wasn't because of anything they'd done. I believed her and hung up the phone.

Now quite frankly, I'm a hard case. And without medication if I function if at all, it's at such a minimal level I'm not much bloody use to anybody. If this was the seventies I'd probably be one of those absentee mothers bombed out on Valium all the time whose husband leaves her for a cheerleader if only to finally get some "perky" into his life. The old school anti-depressants, the tricyclics and MAO inhibitors, had loads of miserable side effects and not many people had the wherewithal to stay on them. The new generation meds are magical by comparison.

What bothers me is the widespread prescribing of antidepressants as a cure all for people who might just be better off exploring the causes of their misery rather than medicating it. If your wife's emotionally abusive it may be time to unload her. If you never admitted to yourself that your entire world view was sculpted by your alcoholic father, it may just be time to go AA. Sometimes pain is telling you that it is time to make some changes in your life, and without it you dwell in a kind of limbo where ideas like *personal growth* don't mean anything at all.

And isn't political growth just an extension of personal growth? If you live in a city like Los Angeles and spend an enormous amount of energy in denial of the fact that the air you're breathing is taking years off your life, isn't it better to confront the problem than to medicate your feelings about it away? If you're tripping over homeless people every time you go below Third Street and it upsets you, isn't that a good thing? Isn't an understanding that in a country with so much wealth virtually everything's become disposable, that to have people sleeping in the street is wrong?

Such a state of affairs is despicable. Noticing how terrible it is, is not mental illness but sanity. Every feeling person knows this. I'm not sure that simply learning to ignore a problem by flooding your neurons with serotonin is an ideal strategy. Maybe political activism to eliminate homelessness makes more sense.

The other thing that bothers me is the assumption seemingly swallowed by Americans at birth, that there are free lunches. It is as universally true as the fact that one and one makes two, that *there are no free lunches, ever*. Anyone who says differently is selling something. If you're psychotic and you take anti-psychotic medication the good news is you'll stop having hallucinations. The bad news is you will walk around feeling like a zombie all day. If you get a liver transplant, the good news is you'll have a functioning liver. The poop end of course, is that you'll have to take anti-rejection meds for the rest of your life, and they will dramatically compromise your immune system. If you run every day for cardiovascular health, eventually your knees will go. If you have your boobs done, the way your ass looks will start to bother you more than your tits ever did. Everything that's worth anything is a trade off: love, family, fast cars, even and especially a warm place to go to the bathroom.

My intuition tells me that anything that effectively treats a condition as devastating as clinical depression will be shown to have a price; and for doctors and pharmaceutical companies to say that it will not smells of snake oil. Truth is, SSRI's haven't been around long enough for anyone to know. Personally I am willing to pay the price. So for all I know my head will blow up when I'm sixty as a result some accumulated critical mass of corkscrewed neurons. This would be a drag but (as Mrs. Thatcher used to say) *there is no alternative*. Not for people like me. The way I look at it, at least I will have had a good time, loved whom I needed to love, and learned to play "Brown Sugar" on the guitar.

But you know, however long I last I'd like to do so with all my mental faculties intact. To this end I have instructed my husband to shoot me if I start to get really squirrelly as a result of corkscrewed neuron syndrome.

I'll have to remember to define the parameters of "squirrelly" to him one of these days.

Me and Doctor Shithead: a Word about Anxiety

The flip side of sadness is fear, but we call it anxiety. Fear sounds too big. Fear is something you have if you're being chased by a lion or the earth starts shaking underneath your feet. Anxiety is less specific, caused by any number of things and usually by all of them combined. Too many near misses on the freeway, too much TV, child rearing, job responsibilities, little things undone that you can't imagine ever having the time to do. Anxiety can be triggered by things barely admitted but right in your face. Things half remembered, suppressed or repressed. Anxiety is walking through a jungle knowing there are trip wires all around, but not being able to see them. Sometimes people get anxiety about having anxiety. This of course, causes more anxiety. It's a cycle that's hard as hell to get out of.

When it got very bad I figured it was only a matter of time before anxiety ate a hole all the way through me. I decided it was time once again, to go see a professional.

Of course it wasn't as simple as that. I belong to an HMO, so I had to get my *primary care physician* to write a referral to a psychiatrist. I didn't think it would be any big deal. I looked a wreck, hadn't slept for days, could barely remember how to spell my name and was doing very disconcerting things like leaving my purse on the roof of the car and driving away, or worse running red lights simply because I didn't notice them.

So I asked my regular doctor, a nice enough guy, but with absolutely no training in mental health, for a referral to a specialist. He assured me he'd write it, but that getting it approved wouldn't be easy. "They hate it when you send these." The way he said "they" gave me the creeps. I felt like I was up against some Orwellian megalith.

So I said to my regular doc, "isn't that what they're there for?" Oh, naive little me. But I'd looked it up in my HMO description of benefits booklet and mental health services were provided for. I didn't understand what the big deal was. If I'd broken my arm *they* wouldn't get upset over a referral to an orthopedic guy.

My doctor didn't argue with me. In fact, I sensed in him a bit of a, *fuck what they want anyway,* attitude. He had been hired as an internist. What was he supposed to do with cases like mine? Still, he warned me again as he wrote out the phone number that what I was asking was non-trivial.

When I got home I called the number. It was some place in San Francisco or Seattle, which I thought a little odd since I live in Arizona. After spending half an hour on hold, someone with a telemarketing license and barely two brain cells to rub together finally took my call. She seemed quite dismayed that I would call The Mental Health Center with a problem concerning my mental health. Finally, after I'd explained my situation—three times using different language each time to say the same thing—she consented to give me a phone number closer to home. I called it. The woman at the other end of the line asked me if I was an immediate threat to myself or others. I said no and she gave me an appointment with a psychiatrist six weeks hence.

It's interesting to note the fundamental disjoint in perception here. Spinning off your rocker is not something you see coming, like with the first sniffles of a cold. It's something you are forced to acknowledge at the point when denying it becomes impossible.

I won't go into what those six weeks were like; it's all hazy anyway, but there were a lot of pills swallowed, chores left undone, traffic violations, and 2:00 AM conversations with the spirits of John Lennon, Napoleon, Edgar Allen Poe, and other insomniac ghosts I've come to know intimately.

Finally the day arrived—my appointment with a genuine psychiatrist, someone who would understand and sympathize with the torment I'd been going through. I walked into his office, a sterile, mid-rate hotel room looking place, decorated with bad Southwestern art: kachinas, glass coyotes, that kind of thing. I was as nervous as a hooker at a VD clinic, sitting on that CostCo couch wondering vaguely whether the walls around me were pink or orange, and how anyone could come up with a color so infuriatingly in between. Eventually, the great man entered. He was in his mid-fifties, shirt and slacks pressed within an inch of their lives. He said hello while flipping through his paperwork and, stroking his iron gray beard and hitching up his pants a time or two, told me he wanted to "send me over to our behavioral health section."

Everything went white. It was like a bad acid flashback. I said, "I thought that's where I was."

He said, "no, no this is our psychiatry department."

"Exactly where I asked Doctor Jumanni to send me," I said.

"Well..." He flipped through more papers, "I think our behavioral health section would be more helpful in this instance. Get you going with some cognitive therapy."

I've got nothing against cognitive therapy—in fact I've had plenty of it—but hearing his words was the equivalent of drowning in high seas and being thrown a loaf of French bread. It's great, I love it. But it didn't have anything to do with my situation.

"I don't think you understand," I told him, and informed him of everything I'd been through in the past six weeks, and several months before. I went into my upbringing, childhood traumas, everything and anything I could think of. And I could not get this guy to actually *hear* me. I was so desperate, I would have taken my clothes off if I thought it would do any good.

"We've got some pretty good people over there," he said, clearly elsewhere, thinking about his acceptance speech at the national psychiatrists' awards, his investment portfolio, his swing, his backhand. Who knows.

So I said, "No, no. I don't think this is something I can talk my way through. I'm too far gone for that."

He flipped through his papers one more time, shook his head in disagreement. "I don't think so."

I couldn't believe it. I could feel my eyes getting hot, tears welling up and underneath it all a feeling of the surreal, like I'd walked into a Salvador Dali painting.

He sighed, audibly, heavily. "Alright," he said as if giving into a small child, "let's say we try a little Prozac."

"What? I told you, I've been on Prozac for eight years. It stopped working. It's all in there." I pointed to the paperwork in his elegantly manicured hands: nails clipped impeccably, not one torn cuticle; unlike mine which looked like I'd had an accident with a meat grinder.

"Hmmmm. Let's try a higher dose then."

Before I could stop him, he was out the door.

He returned with a stack of Prozac sample boxes piled under his chin and proceeded to load them into a white paper bag. For a just an instant, I thought he was going to ask me if I wanted fries with that. "This should last you a good long while. I want you to take forty milligrams a day."

"I don't see why you think that will work any better than what I was taking before," I said.

He looked at me, slightly perplexed, but shook it off, said I'd be amazed what an increased dose could do. Then he said, "I'm going to make you a referral to our behavioral health section. That should help you with the insomnia."

I had my head in my hands, eyes staring at the pristine pink or orange carpet. It matched the walls almost exactly. "How about some sleep meds?"

"Excuse me?" He said, smoothing his pudding bowl haircut.

"Medication, for sleep."

"I don't believe that's indicated with you." And the look on his face said, we both know why, don't we? I didn't understand at all. I wasn't a drug addict. In fact an addictive personality is one of the few problems I don't have.

But what was really funny was the idea that he thought sleeping pills could make me any worse off than I already was. I was literally on the verge of psychosis from not sleeping, fifteen pounds underweight having lost all interest in food, worried about my kids, my marriage, my ability to carry out the simplest routine tasks. My life was literally falling apart as a result of depression and anxiety. The idea that sleeping pills could make things worse seemed beyond absurd. Like that scene in the Monty Python movie, The Life of Brian, when a guard tells a man hollering because he's about to be stoned to death by a mob, that if he doesn't shut up he'll only make things worse for himself. *Worse?* He says incredulously, *how could it be any worse?*

The increased dose of Prozac didn't work, and it would be another eight months before somebody else hit on something that did. But that's not the topper. The topper is that about a week after leaving Doctor Shithead's office, he called me at home and we talked for an hour. I could not get the man off the phone and the dinner I was cooking turned to mush. Confusing, seriously confusing. I mean, when I'd been in his office it was glaringly obvious that he couldn't get rid of me fast enough. Now, here he was hanging on the phone after hours, repeating himself, occasionally even at a loss for words.

Just as the spaghetti on the stovetop began coming apart at a molecular level, it dawned on me what was happening. During my interview, *he'd been looking at someone else's chart.*

Of course he never came right out and said it. But he kept going on about the number of cases he had, how it was hard to keep track of them all, and what a common name mine was. He said sleep medication wasn't indicated for some individuals, but clearly I wasn't one of those people. He told me he thought we should treat both my depression and anxiety aggressively. It was his job, after all, and if we didn't put things on the right track initially, I could call him and—Lord have mercy—if it was under ten minutes, he wouldn't even charge it to my insurance!

He never did get it right. I visited him on six other occasions and with each medication that didn't work, the madder he got. In fact, towards the end I got the distinct impression that he thought I was staying miserable on purpose just to aggravate him.

I wanted to tell him about narcissism, that maybe he should go over to their behavioral health section and get this strange idea that I cared about his caseload or annoyance, talked out. But I knew that would be pointless.

Psychiatry is a weird thing, neither a science nor an art. Because it dwells in this netherworld, people practicing it effectively require a nuanced intelligence that is comparatively rare and frankly, many MD's don't have. The problem with both depression and anxiety disorders is that they impair your critical faculties, so you trust in the system.

But what I discovered is, you can't trust the system. I experienced a fundamental emotional disjoint, a bad vibe if you will, with Dr. Shithead the minute I met him. But my internal dialogue was something along the lines of, *well, the system must know what it's doing.* What I learned is, it doesn't. Clearly there are persons within the system who do, but it's not always easy to find them. Even when you're most depleted, you have to listen to your inner voice. I'm not talking about great enlightened wisdom. Mood disorders render that rare on the ground. I'm talking about the same voice that for example, warns you on the playground, when a creep's lingering too close to your kid. This kind of voice I believe, stays with you as long as you're still breathing.

The trick is in learning to listen for it.

My First Major Depression

It was the climax of a very hard period. When I look back on it, I can clearly recognize a series of events leading up to clinical depression, but in those days, nobody talked about such things and I had nothing to compare my experience to. Like all teenagers, the things happening to me were simply defining life. Teenage is a scary and dangerous time.

I have had my personal history re-written for me more times than a Russian economics textbook. When I mention my teenage years, my mother simply throws up her hands and says, "oh, you were such a nice little girl until you hit puberty..." and to my father's way of thinking, I was just one of those eternal screw ups. Until relatively recently, I've accepted other people's accounts of who I was because I couldn't remember specific things about those years, only a general feeling of chaos and fear. It used to infuriate me when someone would start going on with sweet childhood memories, because I didn't have any. When my most recent major depression came on, my shrink pointed her finger at me and said, "there's the problem."

When I was a kid we didn't have money. My father was an out of work TV writer who, out of financial desperation, became a cop. Unfortunately, I was one of those little girls who dreams of horses. Having one was out of the question—we were nowhere near that economic bracket—though I think I entered every contest there ever was to win a Shetland pony. My parents thought this was pretty funny; I never understood why.

When I was about fourteen, my best friend Tina got a buckskin gelding. I started going to the ranch with her and eventually the lady who ran the place took pity on me and let me start working with a bony, neglected nag called Blue. Blue's owner used to come down about once every three weeks, ride the hell out of the poor beast, then shut her back in her stall where she stood sweating, hoof deep in urine, mud, and manure while slowly dying of worms and neglect.

I started taking her out on the trail: wormed her, brushed her, cleaned up her feet, gave her extra feed. Seattle Slew she was not, but within a couple of months she had put on weight and become a reasonable saddle horse.

None of which her owner knew or cared about. I remember that guy: a squinty, short, blond with an enormous gap between his front teeth, one of those people in which there's something vital missing but you can't quite figure out what. He never seemed to notice that his horse no longer looked like it was going to drop dead under him, but then he wouldn't because his riding style involved going out and buying sharper spurs whenever the poor beast refused to giddy-yap. What he did notice however, was that after about five months in my care, old Blue didn't like him much and decided to buck him off every time he hit the saddle. Everybody thought it was funny, but he got furious because I'd "wrecked" his horse. One day when I rode my bike to the ranch after school, Blue was gone.

I found out where he'd moved her and went over not knowing what I was going to do, only to be met by all five foot-three inches of the owner, and six feet of county sheriff threatening to arrest me if I ever came anywhere near the horse again. It had been raining. I remember the horse standing in six inches of mud inside a stall in which she could barely turn around, looking at me with a tragic mixture of friendship and resignation. I recall feeling like it was me stuck there in the mud; I couldn't even walk over and pat her on the nose and say goodbye. Oh I imagined all kinds of things, like maybe running to the cop, grabbing his pistol and shooting my way out like in a western movie. Jumping on the horse and fleeing into the sunset. But the reality was I fourteen years old. I didn't do anything but walk away. I felt like hell.

This was during the time my friend Tina had figured out the merits of getting really loaded. She showed me how consuming intoxicants, made life feel better. During the next couple of weeks we started drinking tequila and smoking reefer like there was a finite supply we had to get through before either of us saw fifteen. I was the best conduit for both booze and pot, since I had a couple of hippie friends who were over twenty one. But my friend knew some guys who took great pride in being so stoned all the time they could barely stand up. They were into stuff like angel dust, reds, Quaaludes, seconals, and what Tina called muscle relaxers, a.k.a. valium. They could get anything, any time.

I didn't particularly like these drugs, all they did was make me incredibly heavy, stupid, and then unconscious. After a few weeks I could see the lay of the land. The guys scoring them weren't the kind of people you wanted to pass out around, if you catch my drift. Tina and I had a tremendous fight. I wanted to quit the hardcore stoners, she didn't. And they really didn't want to let go of her. She was amazingly beautiful and from their point of view, the more inebriated she was, the better. I remember slapping her trying to get her attention—I'd seen it in a movie—but it didn't work. We didn't see each other so much after that. The days of watching her older brother and his friends lift weights on the patio, and dancing in the living room to her sister's Stones and Beatles records, were over.

But I think the thing that finally got to me was the fallout from my first sexual experience. Oh sure, I'd fooled around some but not actually done the penetration thing, and there was a guy I had a crush on, rode a motorcycle and sneered a lot. One night at a party we did the deed on the mattress of a chaise lounge round the side of the house. I was underwhelmed. As far as I could tell, all it got me was two and a half inches of disappointment, sticky between the legs, and ten of the meanest Mexicans at school wanting to kill me.

Now don't get your knickers in a twist thinking I'm a bigot. I'm not, but in my high school there were white kids and Mexicans. I don't think I even met a black person until I'd graduated high school. White kids and Mexican kids in the San Fernando Valley in the early and mid-seventies hated each other, mostly because while the white kids were kind of this big amorphous blob, all the Mexicans in the school were related to each other. Or said they were. Everybody was somebody's cousin. Being in the minority they'd learned to band together way back in kindergarten. They were really good at it and there was no such thing as having a conflict with only one of them.

Turned out the guy I'd been with was one of theirs. They resolved to kill me. Every damn day I'd have to ditch my last class, or hang around talking to some teacher, then make a break for it when the way looked clear. They cornered me in bathrooms and tried to tear off my clothes, drove by my house screaming obscenities, called the house and hung up repeatedly; there was a big fat one, Alice Morales—humongous hair, a pound of mascara on each eye, who threatened with great regularity to tear my head off. She made stalking me, roughing me up, telling me all the things she and her friends were going to do to me, her life's work. The only reason I didn't die was that one of them had been a friend in elementary school and would tip me off whenever she could, as to where they would be waiting after school. Of course, if I'd been dumb enough not to pay heed, she'd have been obliged to pummel me right along with the rest of them. I knew that.

I used to get a kick out of adults telling me, "kid, you ain't got any problems, enjoy it while you can, you've got it easy." Shit, if this was easy I didn't ever want to know about hard.

This was the point at which I really *discovered* depression. Not in the way a kid discovers that if he mixes vinegar and baking soda, it bubbles. It was not conscious. It was a sort of existential survival strategy. I *knew* these kids at school were going to kill me; and I *knew* since losing Tina, I had no one to turn to. So it occurred to me that if I were already dead, they couldn't kill me.

Throughout the next twenty years—basically until I had kids—I never saw a reason to unload this strategy. Oh, I'd suppressed it, with drugs, sex, studies, and exercise to the point that I sustained injuries that are with me to this day. But problems arose because I'm really bad at faking it. Maybe some people can raise happy kids even if they themselves are miserable. I wasn't one of those people. When my soul dragged me to the edge kicking and screaming, I could finally recognize how dangerous it was out there and do something about it. Being dead in order to live is one of the most bass ackward strategies I have ever heard of, but there's a big difference between logic and psycho-logic. "Psycho logic" is almost a contradiction in terms.

I don't blame the girls at school, or Tina, or teenage, or any of that. As I've gotten older, I've come to understand that we are all the sum total of our experience, and I have no idea whom I would be had my experiences and my reactions to them, been different. I'll tell you one thing though. In looking back, I wish my parents had checked in with me once in awhile. But they didn't. Our family was not that kind. By the time I had reached adolescence, I had already internalized that fact. I try to keep this in mind with my own kids. Best as I can, anyway.

Why it's Okay to Take Medication

If a person is genuinely depressed the greatest gift they can give the people they love is getting treatment. Clinically depressed people are not fun to be around. If they're smart they're relentless downers, inclined to making arguments about why there's no reason to live. In this category you've got your Soren Kierkegaards and Franz Kafkas. On the other hand, if they're not so smart they're inclined to be either abusive substance junkies, acting out when they're loaded, or have tons of psychosomatic illnesses engineered to give them excuses for their unhappiness. "I'd be alright if only I didn't have this chronic back, neck, head, whatever, pain."

I was raised to think doing things for myself was selfish; and quite frankly, that I wasn't worth it anyway. I felt responsible for whatever spiritual pain I did have, and so bound to work it out by myself. Then there was the "tough" problem. Using medication used to be inconsistent with the image I held of myself. I learned a tough persona early on—after all, the best defense really is a good offense—and as far as I was concerned, admitting I wasn't so tough was just flat-out dangerous. I was like Winston Churchill: I would never surrender, only I was my own Nazis.

But then one day out popped this screaming, kicking baby boy. When my first kid was born I looked down there, and laying in a puddle of blood and amniotic fluid was a great big baby with so much strength and life I was absolutely floored. The midwife handed the gooey guy to me; he latched onto a nipple and I swear he hasn't stopped eating since. Most babies have floppy heads. You have to keep a hand on them to support them. Not mine. I half expected him to jump on a Harley-Davidson and haul ass down the road.

I used to go in at night, put my hand on his chest to make sure he was breathing. Having him was like receiving a million dollar income tax refund check from the government. I kept looking heavenward thinking, wait a minute, some mistake has been made. I don't deserve something like this, and I was desperately afraid that the gods would realize their mistake and take him back.

I had to change. It was hard, is hard. It's a continuing project, waking up every morning and re-inventing myself.

A lot of psychologists talk about the fact that depressed people have trouble letting go of their depression. As crazy as this sounds, I think it's true. If you've been depressed for a long time, it defines who you are; so you're not really sure who you'll be without it. I mean think of the writer, poor Franz Kafka. He got famous writing all that dreary existentialist crap about waking up as a giant cockroach, and whatever else. (After that one, I never read anymore. Does anybody?) So the question becomes what would he have been without his misery? Would he have written Hallmark cards? Dime novels about steamy seductions aboard ocean going liners? Would he have deprived the world of all that great literature?

My guess is, no. But his great literature would have been about something other than waking up a giant cockroach. And if he'd never became a famous author? Suppose without his melancholy he had become a juggler, or a musician who never achieved fame, someone we don't know about any more about than the guy who delivered the mail in his neighborhood. Suppose that had been the tradeoff and he would have had some peace?

If you're going to make universal statements, which I am, which I do all the time and it annoys the hell out of some people, but I think everybody would have been better off with the peace. Existence has many dimensions and obsessing about the dark ones invariably produces more darkness.

I agree with Bertrand Russell. He didn't like Frederick Nietzsche's statement, quoted in Conan the Barbarian movies and World Wrestling Federation rings everywhere, *"That which does not kill me makes me stronger."* Horse pucky and double horse pucky. For the most part, suffering just causes despair and out of that comes desperation. Desperate people will do anything. And they do.

I was reading about Robert Downey Jr., wonderful little actor, probably now and forever addicted to drugs and alcohol. I've followed his career for awhile and the one constant is that he keeps trying to destroy himself and failing. Empirically, it would seem that's what he's about; but destroying yourself is a really unnatural thing to do.

Somebody living in his head has clearly got such an agenda however, and he had better evict them soon or they will succeed.

Depressed people are invariably damaged, but the good news is, there is always a seed of who you were before the damage occurred. The trick as an adult is in finding it. I was a smart kid, never thinking the things I was supposed to, about Jesus, my siblings, home, country. And the people I trusted most emotionally pounded me for it. This caused me to turn in on and start feeding on myself. But I was lucky. They didn't get it all. There was some left. As an adult I was able to reconstruct with leftover parts.

Kids come up with some amazing stuff. When my youngest was four we were living in Seattle, very green, lots of ferns. He had always been nuts for dinosaurs—like lots of little boys—and he was staring out the window at some ferns, really concentrating. Suddenly he proclaimed that he had figured out why stegosauruses had bony plates on their backs. (Stegosaurus is the one with the small head, high back covered with flat, bony plates, and narrow tail with the prongs.) Now, I had heard all kinds of theories since he was my second boy child and at that point I had read about eight hundred dinosaur books. Some of them said the plates were for heat radiation. Some of them, that they were defensive. My kid said it was because stegosaurs were green, and with those plates on their backs they could blend in with the ferns when they needed to hide. I have never heard that anywhere before or since.

The point is, most children are smart. They all have an incredible spark unique only to them. Adults unknowingly, and worse sometimes knowingly, stomp it out. Sometimes this is insensitivity. Sometimes it is out of plain old jealousy: they've lost that part of themselves they can't get back, so anyone still hanging on to it makes them mad. Sometimes the stomping, whether from harsh religious values, culture, or even family tradition, is built into whatever philosophy they've consciously or unconsciously, embraced. It all has the same effect.

I've never been convinced that human consciousness of the "I am" variety, is necessarily a good thing. I think it's a by-product of an intense and wholly particular kind of intelligence the human animal possesses, and with certain psychologies, the corollary, "therefore, you are not," is always present. The recipients of this kind of thinking invariably wind up clinically depressed, or with other severe psychological problems.

In the end, I think maybe compassion is of more value than what human beings call intelligence. But it's difficult to be either intelligent or compassionate when you're perennially sad and wounded. In fact, this creates an all encompassing self-absorption. It's hard to get outside yourself when you're in pain. If medication facilitates some relief, how could that be anything other than good?

Narcissism and Depression

There's a connection between narcissism and depression. Virtually everyone in my family suffers from one condition or the other and I don't think it's a coincidence. There's a direct cause and effect relationship.

Contrary to popular belief, narcissists are made and not born. It's one of those vampiric syndromes, like pedophilia. The thing no one ever talks about, but any psychiatrist will tell you, is that successful pedophiles don't simply injure their victims; they turn their victims into other pedophiles. A pedophile doesn't invariably abuse in the physically traumatic sense, but seduces and coerces. Very young children aren't sexual *per se*, but have what I think of as proto-sexuality, and this aspect of their psyches is wired directly into what will later become their sexuality. So sexual stimulation inflicted on a kid often weaves its way into his deep psychic niches and when he gets older, there's a fair chance he's going to be turned on by children or images of sexual situations with children. He may not act on his feelings, but chances are he won't be able to ever entirely vanquish them either. Pete Townshend of The Who is a good example. I do not believe he's a pedophile—nobody can be condemned because of the trauma that happens to lodge in his head—and he's admitted publicly that he was sexually abused. The point is, actions are blameworthy. Thoughts are not. When he was arrested in

London for the child porn thing, he'd obviously slipped. One visit to one Internet site doesn't not a creep make. But he got slammed for it because he showed us something about the human psyche no one wants to look at. As a result, he was nearly ruined.

Instead of getting into their victim's pants, narcissists get into their heads. A little primer on mythology here. Narcissus was a guy who spent all his time staring into a pond at his own reflection. He just couldn't get enough of himself even when a nymph fell in love with him. Oh, part of him wanted to look away and find out who was out there, but he just couldn't. To him, there was simply nothing as compelling as his own reflection.

I've always thought it interesting to contemplate why Narcissus couldn't look away. I mean, most rational people understand that if you're looking at your reflection in a pond, mirror, whatever, and you turn away for a second, you're still there even if your reflection isn't. But poor Narcissus couldn't wrap his mind around this fact. As far as he was concerned, if he couldn't see himself, he'd disappeared.

Which brings me to the very essence of narcissism. Everything in a narcissist's world must be about the narcissist *all the time*, for the simple reason that if it isn't, he believes he'll cease to exist. In a conversation with a narcissist, he will always hijack the content to talk about himself. When a narcissist walks into a party, all heads must turn. When a narcissist is accused of a crime, no matter how heinous, in his mind there are mitigating circumstances which everyone else—cops, attorneys, victims, the general public—are simply too thick to understand. If a narcissist isn't considered smart, beautiful, witty, "special," by everyone in his circle, he will marginalize or otherwise undermine that person, or change circles altogether. Note what I didn't say. Just because someone wants everyone to notice her new dress when she walks into the room, or hairdo, or tattoo, doesn't mean she's a narcissist, just that she's human. *All the time*, are the key words.

Some narcissists isolate themselves but for a small circle of people who can't see through them. They generally have very few true accomplishments to their credit, but spin elaborate fantasies about the person they would be if only the world could finally appreciate their genius. They live in their heads, a lot. These individuals, to their credit, do the least harm for the simple reason that they don't interact with all that many people. It's like a pedophile moving into an exclusive adults-only community. However, these kinds of narcissists sometimes become psychotic. When this happens, all bets are off.

The rest of them are out there. And it's interesting to note that there's also something called—and I'm not making this up—*an inverted narcissist*. An inverted narcissist is someone who only falls in love with narcissists. Maybe this should be called The Echo Syndrome. Hell, I don't know, maybe it is. An inverted narcissist spends his whole life trying to please and/or make the narcissist happy. This is impossible, a Sisyphean task in every sense of the word. Narcissists are never happy. The syndrome doesn't lend itself to happiness. Temporary satisfaction maybe, happiness—never.

Neither is narcissism amenable to cures. When I told my shrink that everyone in my family is a narcissist or a depressive, she told me *I was lucky. Depression can be treated.* Narcissists can never accept that they are the sources of their own hell. The shrink, doctor, psychiatrist, friend, co-worker, has always got it wrong. Oh, they might get it right if they were as smart as he, the narcissist is, but they ain't so they don't. That's the way he sees it. By virtue of who he is, he can't see it any other way.

Right. Back to the part about narcissism being a vampiric syndrome. There are two schools of thought about what kind of parenting creates a narcissistic personality disorder. The first is: the parents loved a child too much: told him he was great even when he wasn't, even when he was, for lack of a better word, shitty. Or maybe they bought him whatever he wanted—expensive toys, clothes, cars, whatever his widdle heart desired. This kind of parenting isn't so much parenting, as paying off a kid to shut him up; and I have no doubt that this kind of behavior towards a child might very well create narcissism. So might lying to him about what he might achieve instead of encouraging him in the things he has a knack for. My sister got really mad at me for telling my kid he wasn't going to grow up to be a professional sax player. Sure, he's good. He won the middle school jazz competition, and was by far the most skilled player in the middle school band. But he was really lazy about practice; I had to harangue him to get an hour out of him four or five days a week. Hell, I know professional musicians who practice eight hours a day and are still starving. Talent is not enough, you have to have a hell of a lot of dedication and a monster work ethic too. What I was telling him was that if he genuinely wanted to be a professional sax player when he was grown, he was going to have to step it up, a lot. In my view, it would have done him a great disservice to tell encourage him otherwise, no matter how good it made him feel. My sister didn't see it that way. She thought I was being unsupportive.

In any case he now practices the electric guitar and bass billions of hours a day. Maybe he'll become a rock star. Maybe I'll finally get that house in Malibu I've always wanted.

The second factor that renders narcissism understandable is that having narcissistic parents is key to becoming a narcissist. A narcissist has to be the center of attention *all the time*, and if you don't pay attention to him he's going to get really angry. Babies are cute and many narcissists have them, not because they know what they're getting into, but because they imagine the kid's going to be an extension of themselves. But even babies are their own people; and normally grow into who they are the same way they grow into adult sized clothes. If they're prevented from doing so by a powerful force, nay not just powerful, *godlike*—which is what a parent is to them—they're going to do one of two things to comply. They're either going to become astoundingly depressed, which was my reaction—if my own father

50

wouldn't allow me to exist, who was I to argue? Or they're going to take the bull by the horns and never trust anyone but themselves to love them properly. That's when they decide to make loving themselves a full time job. No vacation time, no time off, ever. It's a hell of a way to exist.

It's interesting to note that in my experience, if you find a trust fund baby, you won't have to look very far to find a narcissist. It's a million times easier than "Where's Waldo?" Giving your kid enough money to sustain himself for a lifetime is a brilliant strategy for keeping him from ever becoming himself. He will forever be nothing more than a *reflection* of the narcissist. In my opinion this is one of the most sadistic thing you can do to a kid; and I have never met a happy trust fund baby.

The problem with narcissism is that, in the same way that masturbation isn't lovemaking, narcissistic self-love isn't real love. It's a cheap mock-up. Narcissists survive, they don't live.

That's really all I've got to say on the subject, except there's a Brilliant Book by Stephanie Donaldson-Pressman called "The Narcissistic Family." This is the most helpful book on the subject I've ever read.

Low Self Esteem and Basketball

Low self esteem is to depression what a cracked engine block is to a car. It causes the car to break down in the first place then keeps it from getting started again. It's not trivial; it can't be fixed with duct tape. It is essential to the problem. I don't know a lot of depressives who think, as the British so eloquently put it, the sun shines out their arses. I'll even be bold and venture to say that people who genuinely love themselves are not prone to repeated episodes of depression. Depression just isn't structured that way. It is built on a sort of generalized foreboding and internal conviction that fate, while it can be thrown off the scent for a little while, can't be fooled in the long run; and there's not a thing you can do about it.

A group of people I think rates fairly low on the depress-o-meter is professional athletes. There are several reasons for this. By the very nature of their training, athletes' minds and bodies are more integrated than the rest of us. They have to be or they can't perform. This integration is the opposite of the kind of emotional paralysis represented by depression.

(Conversely, at the high end on the depress-o-meter are drunken poets, so desperate to get out of their wretched minds they do things like commit suicide in Hamburg lofts at the age of about twenty one.)

Take the NBA player, Latrell Sprewell. Please. Or that's what his coach P.J. Carlisimo probably said years back when Sprewell tried to strangle him. But that's another story. I was watching an interview with him one afternoon and it occurred to me how professional athletes regularly invoke their mamas. "Moms always said, son, you can do anything you set your mind to. You are a winner. There is nobody as good as you are." I've never heard any of these guys say, "My mama always told me I was a bum and wouldn't amount to nothin." I'll be so bold as to guess that no matter what an individual's inherent talents or abilities, getting that kind of message from someone who's supposed to be on your side would produce, ah... someone who don't amount to nothin'.

A person's self image is shaped by the people around him as he's growing up. If he's given positive messages reinforced with positive action that let him know he's loved, respected and valued, those are the facts he will internalize about himself. There may be other facts too, cultural, social, economic, personal—maybe the kid cheats on his spelling tests, steals food from other people's lunches, whatever. But if a parent can give a child the capacity to believe in himself there is no greater gift.

Allen Iverson, another NBA player, is equally a big pain in the neck. If I was his mom I would have turned him over my knee a long time ago. (Of course then I probably wouldn't be living in a mansion with more rooms than I've had hot lunches.) In any case, nobody would argue that Allen Iverson isn't self-absorbed, (but then he'd have to be.

He's half the size of the rest of the guys out there.) But during the playoffs last year when the camera panned the audience, there was Mom jumping up and down, wearing his number, holding a big sign. Her parenting style—whatever it was—gave him tremendous self- assurance. People might even argue she gave him *too much*, but that little son-of-a-bitch can play.

My hat's off to her. It's an enormous task to give a kid that kind of feeling about himself, especially when he's surrounded by messages every day of his life that he isn't worth anything because he's black, poor, lives on one street rather than another.

I'm not a fortune teller, but I'd be willing to wager that neither Latrell Sprewell nor Allen Iverson will ever suffer chronic depression. Such people may experience episodes of depression due to an illness or injury, rendering them unable to do what they do, but it won't outlast their recovery. Even when the time comes that they can't play anymore, they possess a brand of audacity and egotism can be channeled into something successful simply by virtue of what it is. If you are cocky enough, you can sell socks to double amputees.

I grew up in a lower middle class suburb and the only thing I was ever told about career alternatives, was to get a teaching certificate so I'd have something to fall back on. This to a person who *hated* school. The thought that I was going to graduate only to have to go back—only on the dishing instead of the receiving end—was absolutely horrifying to me. In my mother's own way, I always *got* that this was a sort of anachronistic feminist strategy; this idea that a woman needs a way to make her own money rather than be dependent on a man, or worse, on her back, but the message I internalized was that falling was the best a person like me could ever hope for. Any effort beyond that was ridiculed as hopeless and unrealistic.

To learn to believe in yourself you have to get good at something, to internalize the fact that it's possible, whether it's hockey, the bassoon, algebra. It doesn't matter what it is, but to be informed that who you are has nothing to do with the reality you will eventually inhabit, is crushing.

And when I think about it, of all the teachers I ever had in grade school, I think maybe there were two who were genuinely "called." They were harassed mercilessly by the mediocre, disappointed sluggards who controlled the bureaucracy. In other words, those poor schmucks whose parents had told them the same load of shit mine told me.

I'm not dissing teachers. I'm not even dissing my mother. She is who she is and she kept me from running out into the street and getting hit by a truck. (You might think this is no big deal, but I knew a guy who was one of two out of five kids in one family, who did wander into the street and get hit by trucks. On two separate occasions.) I'm just trying to illustrate the kind of consciousness that unrealistically low expectations create.

If your underlying convictions about the fabric of your very self are negative, if you've molded the idea that you're stupid, unimaginative, slow, incompetent, or unworthy of love into your idea of "self," then chances are you'll be fine as long as nothing rocks the boat. You can go to your nine to five job, have your two point three kids, have sex with your husband or wife and walk your dog. But when something out of the ordinary happens—maybe a death in the family, an economic setback, an extended illness—you will find yourself vulnerable to a kind of sadness so deep there feels like no way you'll ever crawl out of it.

This is called clinical depression. You're not this sad because Grandma died or you got shingles. You're sad because the hounds of hell that have been snapping at your heels for years, are finally breathing down your neck and grabbing hold.

Most people will not admit the depth of the negative feelings they have about themselves to anyone, not even themselves. But if you listen to them talk, the evidence is abundant. I've never quantified it, but off the top of my head I'd say for every fifteen sentences the average woman utters, there will be one or more unwarranted personal criticism. Something about being spaced out, or thick, too short, too tall, or fundamentally incompetent or otherwise lacking in some important way. I notice this particularly in forty-ish women. It's a tendency to overload themselves, and then get self-critical over their inability to handle it all well.

In men there's something different going on that I find disturbing: the willingness to accept themselves as dumb louts. Beer commercials are a particularly good illustration of this: guys sticking their tongues out in phones, slouching around in boxers drooling over near-naked women. Or trying to put something over on the women in their lives simply because it's what guys do. Being a gentleman, of whatever kind, has gone completely out of style. Obviously, this is bad for women, but I think it's bad for men as well. Guys who accept gravitating to their very basest natures make me think I was right when I was eight years old. Boys really are icky.

The idea that it's okay to be a sexist lout is not just demeaning to women; it's destructive to men. No matter what they tell you, men do not just want to get laid. Granted, they do want to get laid, a lot. But they also want what everybody else wants: love, connection, someone to trust with their doubts, fears, and hopes. A guy who tries to live on a steady diet of frat boy nonsense winds up a caricature, a lounge lizard, a car dealer with a bad toupee and eventually, a pathetic old fart making passes at twenty year old waitresses at Denny's.

It used to be very trendy in psychology circles to talk about "human beings" and "human doings." The idea was it was fine to be the former; while being the latter suggested some a sort of hypomanic nutcase. I understand the point. During the eighties and nineties when recreational drugs and booze were becoming less popular—at least within a certain strata of society—being super-busy became the drug of choice. People started running around so much they were exhausting themselves and their families. I felt like a big schlep because I didn't have a high-powered career and four kids, all the while being a supportive wife, on-call chauffer, animal keeper, housekeeper kind of Martha Stewart's latest dessert preparing, woman. Only later did I figure out that no one was handling it. Not even Martha. They just faked it better than I did.

But while simply "being" might have been enough once upon a time, I think even true religious believers are experiencing the sneaking suspicion that maybe just *being* a homo sapien, isn't enough. Spiritually, because of advances in science and research, we've been symbolically knocked out of Heaven and back to hearth. Ninety-nine point four percent of a human being's DNA is the same as a chimpanzee. This fact is some serious shit to think about.

What it means to me is that maybe you have to actually *do* something to get the whole *human thing*, right. Maybe you have to make good ethical choices, make an effort with friendships even though you might not particularly feel like it that day. Learn to play the violin, stop on the way to work and get doughnuts for everybody. Hell, I've known chimpanzees who are better human beings than some human beings.

Maybe you have to dribble the basketball until your arms feel like they're going to fall off, until you can do it in your sleep.

The point for depressives is, doing stuff and taking pride in your accomplishments, isn't about the *stuff*. It's about learning how to admire yourself. If you're at all like me, this is something you didn't learn at your mamas' and daddies' knees.

Art and Depression

According to the Scientific American Book of The Brain, (1999) "Increased rates of suicide, depression and manic-depression among artists have been established by many separate studies. Artists experience up to eighteen times the rate of suicide seen in the general population, eight to ten times the rate of depression and ten to twenty times the rate of manic-depression in its milder form."

Note what this doesn't mean. It does not mean that if you're depressed, you're invariably an artist. It simply means chances are higher that if you are an artist, you do or will suffer from depression at some point.

I've noticed that most scientific books about depression focus on what philosophers call proximate cause. This is a relatively worthless concept most of the time—and the answers it produces are mostly trivial. If a brick falls on my toe, it's obvious that the cause of the pain in my toe is the brick. And I'll be bold here and venture to assert that, without protection (a boot or otherwise thick shoe), any brick falling on any living toe will cause pain. Of course, this information is useless to anyone with an IQ above ten. The relevant question, and the one the average person wants answered is, why did the damn brick fall on my toe? Were the kids playing carelessly, do the bricks need to be restacked? Did I cause it to happen and if so, how can I keep it from happening again?

When it comes to depression, the bricks, according to scientists are low serotonin and norepinephrine levels. Serotonin and norepinephrine are neurotransmitters, the substances that carry messages between the synapses of neurons in the brain. The medical research community thinks that a shortage of these substances causes depression.

This is only vaguely interesting when you're trying to figure out which beam in the house would support your weight should you finally resolve to throw a rope over it. At times like these other, more important questions come to mind. For example, why do I want to throw a rope over the beam in the first place? Or even, are there changes I can make in my life that will eventuate possibilities other that ropes over beams?

The medical community does not know that low serotonin and/or norepinephrine levels cause depression, not in the sense of a falling brick causing broken toes, or any other strong causal sense. A doctor does not take a blood sample and analyze it to determine whether or not you're depressed. What the doctor does know is that often, if you raise serotonin or norepinephrine levels, clinical depression lifts. There is probably a biological mechanism at work here, something more provable than evil spirits, bad karma, or the fact that you neglected to sacrifice a goat at the last full moon, but the medical community does not know what it is.

The problem with scientific, biochemical explanations for depression is that they're almost entirely mechanistic. Psychiatrists commonly confuse proximate cause with true cause (for example, the contractor's dumb-ass assistant stacked the bricks wrong.) I can't tell you the number of these guys who've looked at me like I'm a dumb-ass when I've asked, "yeah, but what causes depression?" Particularly when they've already given me the serotonin, norepinephrine rap. Sometimes, they'll get really desperate and throw in the word "dopamine," which is another neurotransmitter to which the connection to clinical depression has not been established. Usually, they just write me a prescription and chase me out of their offices.

Psychologists, on the other hand, will often tell you depression is caused by psychological traumas that happened when you were small, which will require several years of expensive therapy. If you ask them whether you'll be cured after that, they'll say things like, "that depends on the work you're willing to do," or worse, "that's not up to me." If you're really depressed, this is the point when you leave her office to go find a hosepipe to funnel car exhaust into the front seat of your Toyota. Not only does this person fail to realize that just getting out of bed in the morning is all the work you can manage, but she clearly has no idea as to what depression really is. In other words, she is an insensitive knucklehead.

Which some people are. It doesn't matter how many letters they have after their names. Some of them are born this way—they don't have a lot of awareness about what's really going on around them—and some make themselves this way. Artists are, for the most part, very sensitive individuals. This is a good thing in love, art, poetry and music, but a bad thing in almost any other field. The world is a cold, hard place which would be much colder and harder if everybody was wired like Vincent Van Gogh, Sylvia Plath, or Kurt Cobain. Any one of them would make lousy engineers, cops, surgeons, or paramedics. I'd hate to be badly injured, look up and see Sylvia Plath looking back at me. She'd be too busy feeling my pain to put the splints on! Either that or she wouldn't have come to work in the first place because she was stupefied with a hangover or busy cooking her head in the oven.

The truth is, we live in a tough world and it is painful. Some people simply feel things harder than others. I can sit next to a total stranger in an airport and if he or she is sad, depressed, blue, or simply upset, feel it. I've found this doesn't happen as long as I don't exchange words or make eye contact, but it's a fact about myself I have come to live with; and it's not a quality I want to exterminate. It's the very quality that renders me sensitive to the nuances of human attitude and behavior. In other words, it's one of the qualities that makes me an artist.

If you look at human sensitivity as a continuum, with those who have no empathy for any living thing: psychopaths, serial killers and the like, at one end; saints at the other, it makes sense to supposed that most of us fall in between. Some people are hard asses, and some, for lack of a better description, are soft asses. We bruise easily and often, but if it were not for us, the world would be a sterile, boring place.

So the question for the depressed artist is, should she hold on to her depression for the sake of her art? Will it dull her sensibilities to the degree that she can't produce anything worthwhile.

The answer is no. The only difference in my experience, is that when I'm not depressed, and for me that means on medication, I might sit down next to someone in an airport grieving because his dog's died or his wife has left him, and chances are I will pick up on it. I might even write about what I imagine the guy's experience is, later. What I won't do is get up from my seat when my flight is called, and take that guy's feelings with me. This is a tremendous relief.

I don't think clinical depression is caused by brain chemicals, except in the way that bricks falling on toes cause pain. This makes the point for depressed artists and anyone else interested in holding onto their sensitivity, the restacking of the bricks and taking measures to assure they stay that way. The tricky part comes in learning how to do that for the particular monument, or even simple home, you're looking to construct.

Feeling Jung

Carl Jung was a brilliant man. Unfortunately, anyone trying to get through his writings will conclude he was also a boring man. This is not entirely his fault, and in fact his prose style occasionally waxes lyrical; but when it does he pulls himself up and makes a right turn straight back into tedium. He's forever saying things like, "this experiment proves such and such," or "by our theory we can deduce..." This style seems a little lame now, but during the early part of the twentieth century when he was doing his work, science was held in the thrall of physics. People like Lord Kelvin and Albert Einstein were wowing the world with pithy insights about things that would eventually lead to cool stuff like un-learnable temperature scales and atom bombs.

And so, all of science was held hostage by the rigorous standards of physics until it was discovered that employing such standards, you not only can't do science, you can't do much at all except add two and two.

But even by today's standards psychology ain't a science. To be a science a theory must be able to make predictions. If I say I'm going to mix baking soda and vinegar together, and that when I do it will bubble over, then mix those things together and they bubble over, that's a scientific hypothesis and experiment with positive results. But if I say the reason Jane is neurotic is that she was raised by a neurotic, all that is, is a reasonably good guess.

Making rigorous predictions is impossible in psychology. Oh, you can do a bunch of rat torturing, or if you're with a big important university, monkey torturing, but not much else. Here's why there's a problem. Suppose I have a theory that in human beings depression is caused by environment and not by genetics. To do the experiment, I'd have to separate a pair of identical twins at birth and knowingly send one to a terrible home and the other to a good one. Then at age eighteen or so, I could check back to see which one is miserable and which one isn't. And of course, scientific theories have to be *repeatable,* so a bunch of my colleagues would have to do the same thing in order to see whether my result was a fluke or not. This approach has considerable ethical problems.

Of course the fact that psychology isn't a science does not mean it doesn't have valuable insights, or that it doesn't stumble over the truth sometimes. Jung worked with and helped hundreds of people with mental health problems, and had some damn good insights.

There are a few reasons I like Jungian psychology. One, I've never met a Jungian who tried to sell me something. Two, Jungians are usually fairly gentle, quiet types who don't want to fight, are fairly calm and not doctrinaire. They don't seem to be all that interested in whether they're right, and I've never had one try to make a true believer out of me. This is very different from say, Scientologists, Jehovah's Witnesses, Born-again Christians, and Libertarians.

In itself however, this isn't enough. I've never had an Episcopalian try to convert me, but in that case I think it's more because they don't want people like me in the club. No, the Jungian approach is simply the only one to ever work. And since I didn't start therapy until I was 41—I am now… ah, never mind. The point is I didn't want to spend a lot of time pissing around. I've tried other styles of psychotherapy. There was the guy who put electricity in my ears, and then there was a cognitive lady. She wanted me to explore my role as a woman by doing things like baking cookies more often and going to church. And there was a communist lesbian. What I seem to remember getting from her was that I had good reason to cry since capitalism had so thoroughly screwed me and everybody shackled by the American class system. I'm not sure she was completely wrong, which didn't alter the fact that I was paying her because I wanted to *stop* crying. Who wants to be right when the only alternative it leaves you is suicide?

Nope, to my way of thinking, Jung's the man. Here, I'll lay out his basic tenets in as brief and succinct a manner as possible.

According to Karl Gustav Jung, everybody has two psychological sides, a male and a female. In males the masculine is more fully expressed and in females it's the feminine. Nobody is ever all one or the other.

The anima and animus are the under-expressed parts of the personality. A man has an under-expressed feminine and a woman has an under-expressed masculine. Problems arise when either is excessively repressed.

For example, an intelligent, dynamic woman tells herself she's got a duty to stay at home with the kids, cook the old man dinner, run their social life and liaison with relatives. She does most of the scut work (read, housework). She spends lots of money on makeup and clothes so she'll look like the women on the magazine covers, and let's load the conditions even more, she does look like the women on the magazine covers. She is living her life the way she thinks she is supposed to; doing everything right, fulfilling all the roles society, her church, parents and husband think she should. Yet she's miserable, utterly miserable. What gives?

Herr Doktor would say that of course that's the case. Her animus is completely and utterly repressed.

Before mid adolescence, when her spirit got co-opted by evil forces like the fashion and entertainment industries and the idea that people—particularly men, would like her better if she was dumb—she wanted to be a geologist. A geologist, imagine! What an unfeminine thing to be. Rocks, dirt, math, time periods measured in millions of years. She's all but forgotten about actually wanting to be *something* all those years ago. But Jung would ask, has she forgotten or has she denied her *self* to the degree that her spirit is all but dead?

People trying to kill their own spirits get very depressed. My last big depression started with horrible dreams in which I was controlled and eventually killed by a hung-over looking, sort of Bluto-esque (from the Popeye cartoon), guy. Jung would say my animus was in bad shape. As for the killing and controlling part of the dream, my animus was just going after that blind yet persistent part of me that was trying so hard to be something other than what I am.

I've learned how to get along with my animus better, and when it wants to get my attention it no longer comes to me in dreams as a drunken Bluto, but as a man I admire. Bruce Springsteen pops up periodically. Sting and Michael Jordan used to as well. Sometimes, it was just random, handsome guys from my soap opera. My animus knows how to get my attention.

Once I dreamed of Pee Wee Herman and once of Howard Stern. I chalk those up to bad digestion.

The point is, I try to pay attention. Should I actually have romantic congress with one of these fab guys, it means in my waking life I'm hitting the mark. Maybe I'm working on a piece of writing and have finally gotten it right, or maybe I've got an idea that I need to follow through. It makes sense I think, that if your spirit needs to get your attention, it's going to don a disguise that will grab you, so to speak. Animi aren't dumb, but they don't speak English. They don't yell, "hey knucklehead, pay attention over here."

My shrink tells me the ugly, dark, controlling and deadly man image, is a common one for thirty and forty something women who have yet to find themselves, or have found themselves but lost themselves again.

Men don't have an animus, but rather an anima, an unexpressed feminine. While the ideal woman in this culture is beautiful and about as bright as a twenty-five watt bulb, the ideal man is tall, chiseled of feature, assertive, aggressive, smart, strong and brave. He's not sensitive, kind, weak, passive, contemplative, tolerant, or emotional. Men who possess these qualities are taught to repress them, often with disastrous results, men more so than women because of the unspoken cultural license they're issued at birth to externalize their feelings. Whereas a mentally compromised woman might swallow a bottle of tranquilizers, a man is more likely to beat up his wife, kids, a member of a local minority, or maybe just pick a fight at a bar. You don't get all that many women walking into Burger Kings and spraying bullets everywhere, (Fortunately you don't get all that many men doing it either) but when it happens, it's a man.

A man who won't allow himself to feel is invariably a tyrant. A man who does not acknowledge the fact that he sometimes feels dependant, or nurturing, or tender, or even weak and incompetent, will never figure out how to act like a human being. This is a shame, not just for him but for everybody. It's sad that a man in this culture who can't turn off his feelings is considered a wuss. Think of the many women who find the image of the ultra-masculine, cutthroat corporate executive type, sexy. Hell, they may be from a distance, but I don't think I'd want to get next to one anymore than I would a Rottweiler off the leash.

Jung's theories also offer up an interesting explanation for stalking.

When a part of the personality is thoroughly repressed, it is usually projected onto someone else. Hence we get for example, the overzealous minister's loathing of the libertine, who perceives a drunk to be worse than he actually is, as the result of projecting his own barely restrained demons onto him. Or take an aggressive homophobe's hatred of gays. He's so invested in the idea of male sexuality as a particular thing—something to do with a six-pack, a prostitute and a couple of roofies, perhaps—that whenever he feels anything outside this narrow field, he jumps on it and pushes it down pronto. In this tamped down state, should he encounter the object of his hatred, he's inclined to project all his self-loathing onto him. In a worst case scenario, he calls out the boys and they go out for a night of male bonding and queer stomping. Of course these jerks never really see who they're stomping. He's just some poor victim they've hung their projections on.

In the case of stalking, let's say a guy is in total denial of the feminine. Maybe when he was a kid his father beat him for "being soft," or natural sexual feelings were considered shameful, wrong or dirty. Maybe every time he got attached to an animal it was taken from him, he was ridiculed or worse. Maybe his mother was consistently abused either emotionally or physically. In any case, this guy learns the feminine is dangerous, bad, and to be avoided at all costs.

A man simply cannot survive psychologically this way, any more than a woman can survive psychologically repressing her talents and individuality. So this guy locates his suffocating feminine in someone else, fixating on some Hollywood celebrity perhaps. He sees all her movies, reads everything he can in the magazines about her, but after awhile it isn't enough. He becomes obsessed and directs his energies toward actually finding her. Of course when he does, she tells him to piss off and calls the police, which he interprets as personal rejection. This makes him really mad.

Of course the stalker's obsession has absolutely nothing to do with the actual person who he is stalking. He doesn't see her. All he sees is the image she projects and for whatever reason, it appeals to him. He has no need or desire to know *her* at all. In fact the real woman gets in the way of his delusions.

Big celebrities can hire expensive security firms to keep stalkers away. But other people get stalked pretty often. It happened to me, at least once.

I was working as a waitress and a guy used to come in a lot. After the first couple of times I began asking other people to wait on him, but he kept coming back. Eventually he started following me at night, whether I went to a movie with friends, to a bar, anywhere. It was like a glitch in the Matrix, only there was no Matrix, just this creepy guy. Sometimes, it was almost like seeing a coyote, that is he there or isn't he, thing. Often, I'd think I saw him out of the corner of my eye, but when I looked up he was gone. He never approached me. Until one day.

Pictures started showing up on the windshield of my car, naked women in sexual situations mainly. I told the cops but they said they couldn't do anything. Not until he'd actually done something.

Then one night he followed me home. I lived out in the boonies near San Fernando Valley in Los Angeles, in a trailer on the property of some friends. He came at me, but I out-ran him and I guy I knew chased him off with a shotgun. Luckily, it made an impression, although I still got that "coyote" feeling once in awhile. My boss banned him from the restaurant. That helped.

But some women aren't so lucky. For many this kind of stuff goes on for months or years. Often it's an ex-boyfriend or a husband. But remember, according to Jung's theory, he's not even really after *her*. He's after a part of himself that he's located in her. That's why stalking is so scary. If somebody wants to rob you, you give them what they want and generally, they go away. But if someone's after you for something you simply don't have, and never had in the first place, well it makes for a whole different ballgame.

Any discussion of Jung would be incomplete without mentioning the shadow. The shadow is the part of ourselves we're embarrassed or ashamed about, and it's almost always projected. In extreme cases you get stalkers, the Spanish Inquisition, and the Salem Witch hunts. In less extreme cases you get for example, your Spinster Aunt Betty.

Maybe it goes like this. When Betty was a child and first had sexual feelings—perhaps she was masturbating—her mother caught her and punished her severely. Later when she was older, started getting breasts, her period, turning into a woman, she was bombarded with messages about the carnal and filthy nature of the sex act and everything attached to it. When Betty started dating, she got the indoctrination again and was warned that, "men are only after one thing."

So on a date, maybe with a guy she really likes, he does what guys do—he tries something. Maybe it's something as innocent as an arm around her shoulders, hand holding, a kiss, who knows? Betty freaks out. Mother was right! These evil men creatures are only after one thing. She beats back her date's advances and high tails it home.

But time passes, and the dates go by one by one until she can no longer deny her body's unprompted response to someone's touch. She is horrified, but maybe—like a poor naïf in a nineteen-fifties movie—she gives in to a seductor. Eventually she is so guilt ridden and ashamed, has oppressed and denied her natural sexuality for so long, that it becomes something it wouldn't normally be. Huge and all encompassing. And she projects it on to every man she sees. Men all become sex fiends, *only after one thing.* Mother got it exactly on the nose.

In the sixties and seventies everyone jumped on the bandwagon, agreeing that sexual repression was bad. Well, not everyone but most guys did because they weren't the ones getting pregnant or bad reputations. I remember a few occasions in which I'd say "no," to a guy and he'd sneak in the metaphoric back door by educating me about Sigmund Freud, telling me I really wanted it, that I just didn't know I wanted it. This was all bullshit of course, and afterwards I would discover that no, that wasn't what I had wanted at all.

But even though I and millions of other young girls just like me got suckered by the so-called sexual revolution, by people who used it as means to the very same old ends, I still believe it lifted the lid off the maladaptive sexual attitudes of the fifties.

Any natural human need that is held down artificially pops up somewhere else. It is obvious and ubiquitous. It's why the habitual dieter inevitably sneaks late night gallons of Ben and Jerry's; it's why the celibate priest molests children; it's why the pastors who shout the loudest about sin, are the ones most likely to get caught with hookers. If you pretend a human being is anything other than what he actually is, it creates enormous problems.

When one of my sons wanted to join the Boy Scouts, I was fine with it until I found out they wouldn't allow gay guys to be scoutmasters. To my way of thinking, guess who's more likely to molest a child: an uptight repressed religious zealot who likes to hang out with young boys and lacks the imagination to even ask himself why, or an out of the closet gay man?

It's not even a close call. The repressed guy is the dangerous one, an incident waiting to occur. The other fellow doesn't even make the shortlist.

Heartbroken Kids

I used to have a job where we got dirty and had to take a shower before going home. One afternoon after work, while standing beneath the flow trying to peel the fish scales off my forearm I looked up and saw Liz, a colleague but also a pal, doing the same. I said *hi*, we started gabbing, and when she turned towards the nozzle to wash the soap off her face, I saw a big bite mark on her shoulder. This was no love bite. We're talking bruising, and every tooth save the back molars imprinted well enough to satisfy a forensic pathologist trying to identify a murderer.

It felt too weird to comment on and, well—what does one say? Still, when she started telling me all about her sister visiting from back home, how great it was since she hadn't seen her for five years, I couldn't stand it anymore. "It's a good thing!"

"What?" She gave me a cockeyed look, like I was thoroughly nuts. She was good at that look. The best defense really is a good offence.

"Your shoulder. Is she the one who did that to your shoulder?"

She waved away my concern, the way somebody else might had I commented on a minor scratch. "Oh yeah. We had a fight."

When most people say that, women especially, what they mean is that they had an argument, or maybe they bickered about something. Not Liz, when she fought with her sister they fought like a couple of hyenas over a gazelle shank.

Which left me thinking something I've thought a hundred times before. Human behavior isn't all that complicated. Except of course in our ability to deny the obvious. While I was standing there wondering, and more than a little impressed with the near perfect dentition of sis's teeth (they're from a monied family, it figures), I was spending considerable energy trying to come up with alternate explanations for the obvious. Had Liz had occasion to handle a mature chimpanzee? Could she have had an unfortunate encounter with some kind of an over-bred psychotic dog? But the position of the bite was all wrong. It hadn't been made by something leaping off the ground, but someone coming from above and behind. I guess it was her *big* sister.

But the strange thing was that Liz didn't think it was all that out of the ordinary to be bitten by her sister.

Or then there's Annette, the cowgirl. When I met her she pulled up her shirt to show me the scar where her first husband, housed courtesy of the state these days, had "gutshot her." Then she turned around to show me the scar where her second husband, also residing with the state, had "tried to fillet her." Okay, Annette has rotten taste in men (although people have observed that she may have had it coming. This callous statement outraged my feminist sensibilities at first, but now that I've known her for awhile, I see their point). In any case, what's pertinent is that her brothers, father, and grandfather were also violent people. For Annette, violence is normal.

Maybe if she had a better education—she had almost none—or had spent a significant amount of time around non-violent people—she hasn't—she could have learned that life need not be so rife with trips to the emergency room and near death experiences. But to her, life and violence are inseparable.

Then there's Wynton Marsalis. As far as I know he's never been bitten by a sibling or filleted by a spouse, but he is an awesome trumpet player. The liner notes on a CD state casually that when he was a kid he practiced eight hours a day. What?! Don't kids really want to spend their time skipping, jumping, shooting hoops, and tagging freeway overpasses with spray paint? Apparently not if they're raised in a family where father and brothers are also musicians and think practicing an instrument is a great way to spend all the daylight hours.

I disagree with the notion that what people want is happiness, mostly because I don't see much evidence for it. What they want is what feels normal to them, and when they're adults they strive to create it, even if it endangers their lives. Unfortunately, what's normal isn't usually what's best.

A psychologist told me a story of a woman she counseled who was the victim of tremendous abuse. She'd been shot, punched, thrown out a three story window, raped and sodomized with foreign objects, and knocked out with a baseball bat. (Not all on the same day). Because of her nasty husband, the state had taken her kids away. Yet she continued claiming he was not abusive. Finally, after having all her injuries enumerated for her in grisly detail, she was asked, "how is it that you figure your husband isn't abusive?" Her answer: "he never stabbed me."

Apparently, the home where she grew up was extremely violent, but since Mom wouldn't admit it, neither did the kids. For them violence was something else. Then one day their father stabbed Mom to death and got sent to the Big House. Afterwards they could all point to his crime and say without fear of contradiction, that Dad was a violent man. What made this true? He'd stabbed their mother. So their definition of violence—or unacceptable violence anyway—is somebody who stabs people.

The reasons for depression might seem a little harder to nail down but I don't think they are. In many cases they're just not as obvious. While it's true that some kids are more sensitive than others, it takes several years of abuse or neglect, and sometimes both, to turn what would otherwise be a positive personality trait into something as dysfunctional as clinical depression.

In our culture we have a narrow standard as to what constitutes child abuse or neglect—or at least legally culpable child abuse and neglect. It is almost wholly confined to the physical. Chances are, if you leave you kid alone in his crib all day while you're at work and somebody reports you, the child abuse authorities will come to your house and give you a good dressing down. If you keep doing it (and getting finked on), your kid will eventually wind up in foster care. If you beat your kids and the school nurse, a teacher, or even the bus driver sees evidence for it, chances are fair that once again, provided you keep doing it *and* getting caught, they will also wind up in foster care. But if you feed, clothe, and send your kids to school, you can be the meanest, most thoughtless sonofabitch in the world; you can mess with their heads until the cows come home, *and never get busted for it.*

This is insane. Emotional abuse can and often is just as damaging as physical abuse. And here's a news flash, it can even be more damaging for the simple reason that there is no way to reality check it. The kid might act out at school, bullying other kids, doing poorly on tests, getting "incident reports," getting suspended or even repeatedly expelled, but unless he's got external bruises or wounds of a suspicious nature or comes to school wearing rags, no further investigation will happen. He'll just be labeled "difficult."

Don't misunderstand me. I am not minimizing physical abuse; it is devastating and sometimes fatal. What I'm saying is that if a kid has got a broken arm and a parent is responsible, that parent *may* come under scrutiny. However if a kid is told he's stupid or worthless every day of his life; if he's told he's a fuck up, or unlovable, or ugly, or any number of shitty things *by his parents*, then the fact that that kid is damaged inside, often irreparably, will generally be ignored. A broken arm might get somebody's attention. A broken heart will not.

Yet all the while, even as he's dressed up in his Nike shoes, Guess Jeans, and Armani underpants, even as he's enrolled in a posh school, a cool soccer league, the Boy Scouts, the Mormon Youth, or the most expensive military school in the country, he will be gnawing at himself incessantly from the inside out. He will have internalized the judgments of his parents, and everyone else who has fallen in line with them.

Child abuse and neglect is one of the most insidious and destructive forces in our culture. Broken children grow up to be broken adults and if they don't wind up involved with the criminal justice system, they wind up mixing with everybody else, sometimes in positions of responsibility or power. Of course, these days they don't wait to become adults to express their anger. They march into schools armed with assault weapons.

Every day we all encounter damaged people unknowingly projecting their pain all over the place. Some of them are politicians. Lots of them wind up in the military. These people are often not aware of their pain because, quite frankly, it works for them. Daily, it works to attain short term goals, (mean people may suck, but they also cause others to step out of their way). Sometimes they attain long term goals, like stacking the Supreme Court with morons and bigots.

In the movie Parenthood, the Keanu Reeves character goes on a rant about people needing a license to own a dog, even to catch a fish, but any asshole in the world can have a kid.

I don't believe all you need is love. You also need food, shelter, sex, and a warm place to go to the bathroom. But we could certainly do with a little more love.

My Beef with Philip Larkin

I have a friend who had a vasectomy when he was twenty-one. It took him awhile to find a doctor who would do it, which is completely understandable. Nobody changes his mind more often than wet-behind-the-ears kid.

But my friend wasn't a wet-behind-the-ears kid. He'd had a terrible upbringing, which he just wanted to walk away from with no looking back. He *knew*, and a lot earlier than most people figure it out, that to have a kid would drag him whether he wanted to go or not, back through his own childhood. He made a conscious decision to do something else.

I admire his decision tremendously. Many people have kids anyway and then realize it was a mistake.

Which brings me to Philip Larkin.

THIS BE THE VERSE
(no proclamation intended, it's the name of the poem)
They fuck you up your mum and dad
They may not mean to, but they do.
They'll fill you with the faults they had
Then add some extras, just for you.
But they were fucked up in their time
by fools in old style hats and coats,

who half the time were sloppy stern,
and half at one another's throats.
Man hands misery on to man
it deepens like a coastal shelf
So get out early while you can,
and don't have any kids yourself.

It is a great poem, isn't it? Really seductive in its cynicism. That's the thing with cynicism, it contains a heck of a lot of truth. Sometimes, the kind of truth it might take a psychologist ten years to find.

The problem however, is that Larkin like most poets, is a fatalist. It is simply not the case that because something *did* happen, that it *must continue* to happen. Nor does it mean it was in any way acceptable that it happened in the first place. This is implicit in social policy: if bad things continue happening to particular groups of people, legislation will intervene to stop it. We do not however, apply this logic to childrearing.

It seems like I'm forever hearing, whether someone's done something good or bad, whether he's saved a drowning person or punched out his wife, that "that's how I was raised." My response is, so what? I'm mean, if volition has no part in it, the hero doesn't deserve praise nor the fiend sanction. If we're wholly beings of our upbringing, then nobody has much of a choice. We simply do as we were programmed to do.

Of course I know this is just a particular way of talking: giving kudos to Ma and Pa, or whatever. But suppose your parents didn't raise you to be a hero? Suppose, consciously or unconsciously, they raised you to be a shit? Are you going to be a shit to your own kid because that's the way you were raised? I think if you were abused and refuse to acknowledge it, then the answer is yes.

If you were abused as a kid and have elected to pretend it is other than what it was, you will invariably inflict your pain on your kids. Larkin is right: misery does beget misery, unless an individual is prepared to look at the reality of his upbringing.

Now is when people generally shake their heads. They say, "no, my dad was a tough guy; and I swore I'd never lay a hand on my kids. End of story."

Well, hold that bus.

The human psyche is a tricky and determined thing. You have to actually make amends with it in order for it to fall into line. Failing to recognize a brutal upbringing for what it was is like telling the psyche, "okay, I'm sorry, but you know you brought it on yourself." The psychic response is going to be "oh well, fuck you then," figuratively speaking, and the damaged psyche will carry on with its agenda behind your back. Your psyche is way smarter than you are.

This is where emotional abuse starts. Here's an example of what I mean.

When one of my kids was about three, I was teaching him to ride a tricycle. We didn't have any sidewalks in our neighborhood; it was a quiet residential street, relatively safe. As I stood on the outside trying to keep him out of the traffic lane, he kept veering off there anyway. Every damn time I'd scoot him back toward the curb, he'd point the thing the other way. I kept saying, "don't head out into traffic, don't turn the wheel," over and over and he wouldn't listen. I wasn't using abusive language, wasn't calling him names. I'm naturally careful of the words I choose. But I could hear my tone of voice, and heard what I must have sounded like to him. I was saying, "don't head into traffic," but the tone of my voice was exactly the same one my father used on me. It said, "you dope! I'm so exasperated. Why did I have to have such a thick kid anyway? Stupid, stupid, stupid."

And when I was small, I had reacted exactly the same way my son was reacting in that moment. The more I talked, the more he did the exact opposite of what I wanted. When someone is talking to you like you're an idiot, complying with instructions seems to make them right. Or maybe in not complying, a child imagines he's giving the adult what he wants. I don't know. I still don't understand the logic of it; but am sure this kind of behavior elicited beatings somewhere along my lineage and maybe not so far back. My father translated it into emotional abuse and at that moment, so was I.

The realization that even with all the parenting books I'd read, even with the intensity of love that I felt for my son, I was still capable of sounding like an absolute shit, told me I had a lot more work to do before I could actually be the good parent I wanted to be. I would have to reach miles beyond my experience to get what I needed. Miles and miles.

Several years ago it was very trendy to *forgive* your parents by acknowledging *that they were doing the best they could at that time with the resources available to them.* It seemed like every new-agey type I encountered, was walking around spouting this stuff in an attempt to encompass everything from forgotten birthdays to rape. While this approach might have worked with the former, I'm sure many individuals experienced in things more akin to the latter, were positively brutalized by it.

The truth is, some things actually are unforgivable. Maybe you have to cope, maybe you just have to put the anger down because it's tearing you up inside. Maybe you even have to castigate. But "forgiveness?" That's all fine for pop psychology, but brutes and criminals have kids too and it's unrealistic for people with minor injuries to go around telling the less lucky they're lacking somehow because they can't forgive.

This is where Larkin's poem comes in. When this realization occurs, it's tempting to feel the victim of fate, to be overwhelmed imagining all the pain through all the generations, and to see it as something as layered and every bit as solid as Larkin's coastal shelf. It makes you want to cry for your father and mother, and all of your ancestors back through time. It breeds an existential resignation. This is a terrible place from which to become a parent.

Regarding the bike experience, the moment I realized I was being nasty to my three year old it became my responsibility to *stop doing that*. The fact that in my families' history, that sort of thing is built in, had nothing to do with the decision I had to make. Realization entails responsibility. This is basic and you don't have to have a psychology degree to figure it out. You do however, require a grip on reality. Sometimes this involves admitting some nasty truths. It can be absolutely terrifying. Until you come to recognize that the past is finished. The only way it can get you is if you refuse to stand up to it.

Quick Fixes

There are no such things as quick fixes for psychic pain, but no one wants to believe that. When I was young I sure as hell didn't, and in Southern California, I didn't have to. Eastern mysticism and gurus were all the thing in the seventies. But when I looked east it didn't look so great to me.

There are two places in the world I've never wanted to visit. One is China and the other is India. India looks crowded, dirty, and poor. If that's enlightenment they can keep it. Loads of my hippie friends were always talking about Gandhi as some kind of role model and while I can see there was plenty of good in the man, he also used to sleep bundled up with adolescent girls in order to challenge his capacity for sexual abstinence. Since I was an adolescent girl and already sick to death of the type, it made him look like just another old pervert to me.

When it comes to holy men, I still say now exactly what I said then: to hell with them. They're always going out wandering in the desert, renouncing worldliness, and seeking enlightenment; and my question is, what happened to the Mrs. and the kids after the old man (of whatever creed) buggered off? I mean, if a holy man has to renounce something, it's reasonable to expect that previously he indulged in it freely. Saint Augustine even admits this in his Confessions "Lord make me chaste, but not yet." Well, I assume that since there being no reliable means of birth control in his day, his lack of chastity affected plenty of people. From what I have read, old Augustine was not only married but knew every hooker in the neighborhood on a first name basis. So what did all the Mrs. Holy men do when their old men went out to wander and pray for twenty years? My guess is that they were left with nothing but a few pair of breasts and a smile.

You can keep every damn one of your holy men. And you can bet that if anyone holy ever does arrive, it's going to be a woman.

When I was a kid there was a guy we used to call "The Squat Guru." He was a fat, teenage East Indian forever surrounded by a bevy of beach girls, who took his entourage of ten Rolls Royce's along wherever he went. I always figured the girl thing was kind of Gandhi-esque, meaning he was challenging his willpower. I never understood the car thing, however. I asked one of his devotees about it, said "if he's so holy how come he's got so many cars? He could feed all of South India with the money it took to buy those cars." The devotee looked at me with serenely and said, "because he can."

I didn't know what that meant then and I still don't.

Ah, the good old days. There were so many people sticking, "ananda's" at the end of their names and charging five-hundred dollars a pop for weekend enlightenment seminars. Someone took me to see an old lady guru once. She squinted, petted my dog, and told me I was old enough to start shaving my legs. Next!

These days I think all the clubs have to do with Jesus. Anandas one day, Jesus the next. It's all the same to me.

And let's not forget about EST, and all the sons of EST. My older sister talked me into taking something called Lifespring. She was absolutely fanatical about it, thought it would fix me, and was convinced it had fixed her. It was *the answer*, and since she wasn't generally into the consciousness raising thing and offered to pay for it, I could hardly say no. At least there weren't any gurus involved. I was about twenty or twenty-one and had a reasonable job at the time so I gathered the money myself and trotted off.

It was one of those Thursday, Friday afternoon, all day Saturday and Sunday things. I was working in Palos Verdes and had to drive into Glendale for it—about an hours drive, hour and a half if the traffic was bad—but hey, she said it was going to change my life and so did everyone at the free introductory lecture. The free introductory lecture was one of those events where you say, "I dunno—five hundred dollars is kind of a lot," and whatever acolyte you are talking to just laughs, like questioning the cost for such a extraordinarily blessing is about as absurd as a Rabbi in charge of the Vatican. Then they give you one of those inclusive grins that says *you'll understand soon!* I imagine it was the kind of grin Jim Jones had on his face while deciding which flavor of Kool-Aid to mix up.

It took place in a big room with a stage, must have been two-hundred or so people there at my "training." One of their primary rules was that you couldn't leave the room except for scheduled breaks, and they had thugs dressed in suits stationed at all the doors to make sure you didn't. We would do group activities, things like picking the ugliest person in the group and telling him what was so objectionable about him. I guess this was preparation in case any of us wanted to join a lynch mob. I remember another exercise in which you partnered up with someone and screamed, "what do you want?" in her face for about ten minutes. I teamed up with my younger sister who had joined in, and we got yelled at for messing around. She'd yell, "What do you want?" And I'd scream, "I want you to stop screaming in my face." "What do you want?" "I want to go take a nap." "What do you want?" "I want to go take a pee." After that they wouldn't let us partner anymore. We were acting childishly. I remember surprisingly little of it all now. Probably because early on Sunday morning, I started barfing.

I had felt a little nauseated the night before but chocked it up to greasy food. Sunday morning at the training however, it was coming on strong. I was pretty intimidated by the guards at all the doors, not just because they looked strong, but they had that squeaky clean look that makes people like me feel guilty for breathing, like well manicured robots, you know? Superior yet understanding in the indulgent manner of a kindly executioner upon your requesting a fresh edge on that over-used axe. And they all looked about six foot-ten. I'm fairly tall but I had to look way up.

But the point came when I had to get out of that room. I couldn't concentrate on anything the trainers were saying anyway. I told a big woman in a tight linen skirt that I had to get out, but she just looked at her partner knowingly and told me break was in a little while. I told her I had to get out now, and she started to say something else but relented when I began heaving in her direction. She sprang that door faster than you could say Jan Michael Vincent. I just made it to a garbage can in the hallway.

I went back into the room and for such enlightened people, those guards gave me some pretty nasty looks—which didn't stop me from having to exit every half hour for the next two hours.

When break finally came, the lead trainer took me outside and sat me down for a little talk. He told me I was disrupting the training, and that the reason I was doing so was that my subconscious was looking for a way out of facing whatever the training was bringing me to. He said I needed to quit the puking and surrender. I panicked. There were loads of people by this point who were standing up, admitting for the first time that their father had raped them, or they'd seen their drunken mother strangle the cat when they were four. I was wondering how many rapes and cat-stranglings I was repressing, and was altogether terrified by the power of my subconscious. Wow! There was something so terrifying I'd rather puke my guts out than look at. To my way of thinking, I was more screwed than even I thought I was. This turned out to be right in the end.

Acting's all in the eyes they say, but it's also in the hair—this trainer's was not gray, but silver and perfect, not a single one out of place. His suit was a sort of high-gray color which complemented his hair color and sky-blue eyes like a piano with a classical guitar. I've never seen a jaw so squared or nose so straight. He was like some sort of weekend-seminar god and he was getting to me. I struggled to make something up—just to get away from the glow of this great man's presence—when I said excuse me, leaned over and puked into a potted bougainvillea.

I did last the day though. When the lunch break came, I went and took a nap in my car and later on, though I felt like retching a time or two, the well was dry and I was able to relax a little. That slick gray trainer kept giving me the stink-eye. One thing about these people with their shit all together, they never have much sense of humor.

The next day a guy I'd met once over the weekend called me at my little duplex home in San Pedro. After the seminar we had all been assigned a sort of minder, someone to talk us into coming to the next seminar, which was a thousand dollars. He kept telling me how worth it, it was. Look how it had changed *his* life, after all! His brother had been killed in Vietnam, his mother had died of breast cancer and his father, so grief addled he couldn't work and make the mortgage payment anymore, had just been forced to accept foreclosure on the family home. Hey, this guy, my minder, didn't feel a thing. Lifespring had done this for him. Here it was, ostensibly the worst time in his entire life and he felt great. Wasn't that kind of peace worth a measly thousand dollars?

I sat on the floor, phone to my ear half listening and started thumbing through my checkbook. I was trying to remember whether I'd paid the electric bill, and when I glanced at the calendar on the top flap—the place where I marked the dates of my menstrual periods—I noticed a long blank period. Oh shit. The mysterious upchucking at the seminar wasn't mysterious anymore.

I made my excuses to the minder, and the next day when he called again to get my down payment, told him I was busy.

The whole Lifespring experience drove home a very significant lesson for me. Psychic pain takes a long time to build to the point in which it cripples your life. It just plain doesn't make sense to think it can be remedied in a weekend, a week, or even a year. It's not convenient to see things this way, nor is the prospect of slogging back through all the shit, pleasant. It is however, reality. You can fling yourself against it until you break, or choose to work with it.

Buddhism and Fibromyalgia

I had a college professor once, Buddhism; I don't even remember his name. I don't remember much of what he said either, because his Japanese accent was so thick I couldn't understand him. He'd been hired to teach a low level class; and I think almost everyone did final papers on Zen, attempting to answer the question, what is the sound of one student flunking? If a student flunks in the forest and no one's there to hear him, does he still flunk? But this prof was a good guy. He knew he mostly wasn't connecting and gave everybody except the most egregious dummies "B's," erring on the side of caution.

But there was one story he told in surprisingly clear tones. Maybe it was his presentation, the eerie way he ceased being a middle aged college professor and slipped almost effortlessly into being a little kid in post war Japan.

He said as soon as the war ended he was walking through a field, vaguely aware of the national mood—one of disgrace and sadness. But he was just a little kid, glad the war was over and everyone could be friends again. The sun was shining, the field was damp from the previous night's rain and just as he started hurrying to keep from getting his shoes wet, he looked up and saw an American plane. "I was so happy, war over, so I look up and wave, like this." He waved his hand back and forth the way all seven year olds do, without worrying whether it will be returned, without thinking at all, just feeling good. The pilot of the plane started shooting at him.

When he got to this point in the story he put his hands on the side of his head, covering his ears like he couldn't bear to hear, yet was trying to hold his head together at the same time. It was obvious that in the telling, he was living that morning all over again. I could see the field, the little boy, the plane. I could feel his shock and complete bewilderment. It was one of those moments of such acutely clear human communication it makes you believe telepathy is real.

I remember virtually nothing else about the class, except that I got a "B," and what he said when he took his hands off his head. "It's not just me, you live out there, you all crazy." And he pointed out the window. He didn't mean in a field, or in Japan. He meant out there in the world.

Loads of people say they're crazy but they don't mean it. It's like those dopey signs, "You don't have to be crazy to work here, but it helps." They mean zany, wacky, maybe a wee bit neurotic, but nothing above the radar is what they mean. Something like quirky.

Because admitting you're crazy and really meaning crazy is dangerous. People will cross the street to avoid you. Every time they talk to you the conversation will carry the caveat, *I can discount them, even if what they say is true because after all, they're crazy.*

Well, I'm a little crazy, but not dangerous. Thanks to the Buddhism professor for letting me know I'm not alone.

Because he's right. Life drives you crazy and it doesn't take a major event like being shot at from a plane. When I think about enlightenment I don't think of it as some pie-in-the-sky journey to the light. I think of it as a journey from nuts to sanity. I think we'd all be a lot better off if everybody would be like the Buddhism professor and just admit they are nuts. Then maybe life would be neater, like arithmetic. If you add 7+4 and get 12, then 12 to 2 and get 14, then add them all together, you're going to get 25 which is the wrong answer. The right answer is 24, but you're never going to get it unless you go back and correct the first part of the problem. *Being nuts is the first part of the human problem.*

An old friend of mine called me a few months ago. She was thinking of killing herself because she's in so much pain from fibromyalgia, that she can't take it anymore. She's exhausted all the time but can't sleep, has terrible stomach problems, says she feels like she's been stabbed with knives forty-seven times. She admitted she was depressed, but won't take anti-depressants because they make her head buzz.

Now my concern obviously, was in talking her out of it. I couldn't rush over there—she lives six hundred miles away. I mustered everything I knew about talking suicidal people down. I don't even know where I learned it. TV? The child abuse hotline I worked for? But wait. Those people mostly wanted to kill their kids, not themselves. I just hung on the phone for a couple of hours and let her talk. We reminisced about shit we got up to when we were young, and at the end of the phone call her voice sounded clearer and she said she felt better. I told her I'd call her in the morning at ten and she made me promise five times. I put a big note on my computer screen, wrote it on my hand, told my kids to remind me. I had it covered.

At the time, I didn't know much about fibromyalgia, but when I did some research, found out it's not a clear cut thing. People who have it—ninety percent of whom are women—suffer enormously, mainly with diffuse and chronic muscle pain. The problem is that when they're physically examined there is no evidence of muscle inflammation, nor anything detectable in lab tests or X-rays. There is no pathology revealed in tissue biopsies. In short, some doctors tell women so debilitated they can do nothing but lay in bed, that it's all in their heads. Which is of course tantamount to telling them they're nuts.

If forced to pick one adjective people have forever used to describe my friend, it's *nuts*. Since the day I met her in the third grade she's been given to temper tantrums and extreme mood swings. At twelve or thirteen when everybody else was getting high, smoking a little weed, that kind of thing, she was swallowing palmfuls of seconals and chasing them with vodka. She's been emotionally unstable and self-destructive since the day that I met her.

So I shouldn't have been surprised when, after our phone call the next day, she sent me a scathing letter for finally suggesting what I'd thought privately for years. That her depression and mood swings were a major problem and should be treated aggressively. She told me to mind my own business because I don't understand her disease, and no one could advise her about anything who hadn't been through it. She accused me of attacking her by inferring the problem is all in her head.

Now at the time, I didn't know the difference between fibromyalgia and tuberculosis. She told me it was a disease, I assumed she'd been afflicted with a terrible physical disease. It could have been the same thing as tetanus for all I knew. I just did what you do when someone's suicidal, I tried to talk her out of it.

I still don't know what causes fibromyalgia. For all I know it could be anything from a pepper allergy to something neurological nobody understands yet. But what I do know is that even if it were something psychogenic—psychologically and not physiologically caused—it wouldn't mean it doesn't exist and that the pain isn't real. Someone try telling Karen Carpenter's family that anorexia, which is clearly a *nut disease* (can I get an "amen" for the new nomenclature), isn't fatal.

I wonder what would happen if someone with fibromyalgia stood up and said, "I'm in so much deep and persistent psychic pain that I am physicalizing it." I'm not saying that would cure it, but it might at least create an inroad worth looking at. What would happen if someone with anorexia stood up before an international conference of fashion designers, Cosmopolitan Magazine, and their obsessive compulsive parents and said "I feel so inadequate I'm starving myself to death."

I attribute a lot of these afflictions to Rene Descartes and his codifying of the mind/body split. That guy's got a lot to answer for. Have you ever noticed that when you throw a green log on a fire it hisses? Rene Descartes, the father of modern rationalism, noticed it too and figured, correctly, that the hissing was the result of a natural physical process i.e. the out-gassing of the oxygen in the wood. This led him to conclude that if you threw a cat on a fire, for example, the noise it makes is for the same reason. It couldn't be pain, because to feel pain you have to have a soul, and to have a soul you have to think in a particularly cognitive way. I don't know how many cats M. Descartes threw on fires, but clearly by his definition, if he had been inclined to, it wouldn't have been a problem. I like to remember these things. They help keep the inherent cruelty of human reasoning in perspective.

The mind and the body are not separate things. Ask any professional musician. Piano players particularly, will acknowledge that fingers learn entire arpeggios that if intruded upon by conscious thought midway through, are ruined. The discipline comes in the musician knowing when not to think intrusively and to let his fingers do what they have learned. I've found this with my own guitar playing. Sometimes I'll sit down to play something and if I can quiet my mind, my physical memory of the song eventually returns. Human beings are not robots like my son's toys in which something in the head makes the body move. I'd argue it's just the opposite. The body makes the head move.

People are who they are for specific reasons; and they carry the record of their experiences in every cell. The body remembers emotional, sexual, or physical abuse even if the head blocks it out for its own reasons. The body sends signals all the time: "don't do that, it makes me nervous; do this or you'll get a stomach ache; don't go out with that guy, he's a creep; hey you, I'm giving you a rash to get your attention and all you're going to do is put cortisone cream on it? Hello! Body to brain, body to brain... is anyone listening out there?" These messages are encoded in our ways of speaking: such and such is a pain in the neck, that guy over there is a pain in the ass. The problem is we don't listen. Finally, in the case of depression, maybe your body is going to keep you awake until you consent to learn just one single lesson about reality instead of whatever lies or delusions are knocking around in your head. Or maybe it's going to keep you in bed because your neuroses and obsessions are so fucking exhausting. I don't know what fibromyalgia is saying; I'm only saying it's worth asking it.

There are many people willing to crucify themselves on the cross of their belief systems rather than face the truth—uncomfortable, frightening truths like someone you love betrayed you, someone who's love you needed really didn't care much at all, someone who was supposed to protect you exploited you instead. This is hard shit to face, but just because you can't or won't take the time to see it doesn't mean it isn't there. Your body knows what's real, and if you don't listen to it whisper, it will start screaming.

How far do I want to take this? I don't know—cancer, death?

There have certainly been cases of people willing themselves to die. Have you ever tried to starve yourself to death? It's hard. I miss lunch and I'm yowling, yet half the people in US Magazine are making careers out of it. I would argue that all the pain, grief, and violence in our world is the physical manifestation of otherwise unexpressed psychic pain.

So would the Buddhists. Maybe that professor did get through to me after all.

Insomnia

When I had my first major depression, insomnia augured it in with a ten day stretch of wakefulness so severe, I thought I was going to die. Not that all depressives are insomniacs, nor are all insomniacs depressives. Lots of things can cause periodic insomnia including too much caffeine, transient anxiety, or hormonal changes. Drinking too much wine can cause some to awaken at three or so in the morning, and not be able to get back to sleep.

Those are the easy ones. Insomnia can also signify anxiety disorders, bi-polar illness, and neurological problems. With some individuals it marks major depression, and is worth mentioning because insomnia-caused depression fools a lot of people. The tendency is to focus on the sleep problem, then start telling yourself that everything would be okay, if only you could get some sleep.

This is not true. What you actually need is treatment for the depression. Depression can be a tricky bastard. It doesn't want to be found out, because in our culture, it is looked upon not so much as a mental illness, but as a moral failing. This is still true and with people who have been raised with a "stiff upper lip" mentality, being burned out from lack of sleep is somehow more acceptable than the sin of falling in on yourself. I think a lot of people are more willing to allow themselves to be insomniacs than they are to admitting clinical depression.

The first time I had insomnia it was an ordeal the likes of which I hope I never have to experience again. Night after night I couldn't sleep. I remember one night of wakefulness, after about four, that awful feeling, a buzzing in the blood. Someone had given me a joint, which had been sitting in my jewelry box for over a year, and though I smoked it the buzzing remained. It wasn't dulled a smidge, though it did acquire a sort of surreal, Bill and Ted aspect. Then I drank a tumbler of whisky. Nothing, absolutely nothing. Like shooting a water pistol at a forest fire.

The next night at four o'clock in the morning, I got out of bed and went for a forty mile bike ride, figuring I could pedal my way to physical exhaustion. Wrong again. All I did was pump my way into a sort of psychotic awareness of color and the dangerous edges of the things all around me. That's what lack of sleep does. It removes all the padding until wakefulness becomes unbearable. Everything you see, hear, and touch turns spiky and jagged; everything you try to understand becomes incomprehensible. Prolonged insomnia renders you unable to do anything except obsess about the insomnia. It's terrifying, and to this day insomnia still frightens me.

However with practice, I've gotten better at handling it and have even learned to recognize depression insomnia from garden variety stress insomnia. Of course these days, owing to peri-menopause, the gods in their infinite wisdom have seen fit to give me a new kind of insomnia. You guessed it, peri-menopausal insomnia. Are these guys kind, or what? When this happens I say to hell with it, and take a pill. It seems to go away once I get my period.

Maternal insomnia is also worth a mention. I, like many women, am fiercely maternal. I've adopted everything from stray kittens to wounded pigeons as far back as I can remember. When I had my first kid, this tendency launched itself into a whole new orbit and if my infant grunted, sighed, kicked off a blanket or did virtually anything, I awoke. This didn't stop when we moved him to another room. My hearing simply got better. After awhile, I began sleeping so lightly it was tantamount to not sleeping at all. This tendency has never completely left me. I know this exists in other women because they've told me; and I've even met a man or two who recognize it. This kind of insomnia, when combined with the other stresses of becoming a new parent, can lead to major depressive events. This is different from post-partum depression, the hormonal let-down many women have after giving birth, and both the insomnia and the depression must be addressed before they become habitual. Trust me on this one.

I was up in the night once, lying on the front walk watching a meteor shower around one thirty or two in the morning. Man I was tired, past the point of being fed up, or angry, past the point of feeling anything at all, just focused on how beautiful the night sky is. We live on the edge of a medium sized city and unlike Los Angeles, where we used to live, you can see the stars here. I was okay until I started thinking about my friends and neighbors sleeping blissfully in their beds. I got myself all worked up, imagined floating into their bedrooms on my cloud of wakefulness and disconnected sensibilities, and biting them right in their lily white throats. I understand where vampire myths come from now. You get mad when everyone is sleeping and you're not.

But, when you get in into perspective, when all is said and done, there are worse things than not sleeping at night. Flesh-eating bacteria and malaria, for example, are far worse, as are amoebic dysentery and spinal meningitis. I'd come up with more, but gimme a break. I'm working on two hours sleep here.

Big Mac Aversion Disorder

Sitting in a desert cafe, beautiful, hummingbird vines climbing up wooden trellises, mesquite and palo verde trees shading a patio area staffed with young, nubile servers taking care of customer's needs professionally yet subtly. There's a gentle breeze blowing from the west, the smell of basil coming from the kitchen. I'm waiting for my friend Fiona, who's always busy. It's an honor she's agreed to meet me at all and I'm thrilled when her lithe form saunters in and she plants her fanny opposite mine. I understand, of course, *what with the bloody kids—Remy and his oboe, and little Chelsea playing Clytemnestra in front of all those people in the school play*, that time is a spare commodity in Fiona's world. She starts complaining immediately, says she never knew she'd have a second career as a bloody taxi driver. I understand; I have to, especially after she proclaims there's something *wrong* with people who don't understand.

Now the thing about Fiona, she's elevated misery to an art form; and if everybody else would pay the kind of proper attention to life's details that she does, they'd be miserable too. They're just not getting it right, damnit! I had made the mistake a year of two earlier of telling her I was on Prozac. I remember the way she looked at me with great pity, like I'd just told her both my kidneys were failing.

The waiter comes up, we order herb tea. She's a no-caffeine, vegetarian kind o' gal, Fiona.

When the server walks away, she broadsides me. "Are you still taking the bloody Prozac?"

As it happened, that month I was experimenting with going off it; it was not going particularly well. "Oh, that stuff? No."

"That's good. Silly bloody idea, that. They're always pushing pills on you, aren't they?"

I'm not sure whether she means me, or if she means, we. "There is a pill for everything," I say, a little hesitantly.

"One of them tried to give me sodding pills. They don't understand, these American doctors; we don't all think like they do." She shakes her head in an unmistakable gesture of English desperation. I still don't know if she's talking about *me* or *we* as in *us*. Now I've got to figure out if she means *they—Americans* or *they—doctors*. And it's quite possible if it's the former, we're no longer talking about me or we, but *her.*

"That's true," I'm so confused, and I'll admit, wimpy. The English intimidate me, at least the posh ones do.

"One of these days they'll have pills for people who don't like Big Macs!"

This is how people like Fiona trip people like me up. I happen to believe they will have a pill one day for people who don't like Big Macs. I also believe they'll have a mental disease called "Big Mac Aversion Disorder," and they will advertise pills to cure it during afternoon talk shows and soap operas. They'll show a scene during the commercial depicting a bunch of attractive, laughing people bonding over hamburgers, while the Aversion Disordered person presses her nose against the window looking forlorn and alienated. However, and this is a big however, this doesn't mean that Big Mac Aversion Disorder is anything like clinical depression, or that the pill for it will be anything like Prozac or any of the others. As far as I know, there are no statistics indicating the dislike of Big Macs is life threatening.

But like I said, I'm afraid of the English; and I laugh at her Big Mac crack. Fiona's pretty funny sometimes, whether she's trying to be or not.

She reaches across the table, puts her hand on mine and knits her brow in compassion, like she wants to make me a cup of tea. "And we all know that it's not you, it's this bloody place."

I moved to this town with my old man when he got a job here. If given a choice, it's not first on my list of settling down places, and Fiona knows it. "Ralph Waldo Emerson said it's the geography of the heart that matters," I mumble lamely.

Fiona makes a brush-off motion with her hand and rolls her eyes. She doesn't have to say a thing. And the truth is, I've wondered about that statement too. Yeah, if you've got deep pain in your heart, whether you're living in a trailer in Yuma or a beach house in Malibu, you're still going to have it. But as far as learning to get over it, my money's on the guy with the beach house in Malibu. For the guy in the trailer in Yuma, nothing short of a Buddha-like detachment is going to do the trick.

Throughout the rest of the meal, Fiona tells me about her life, about her worthless husband who won't help with the kids, the worthless school women who won't sit the chess club, the worthless US postal service and the bloody worthless UPS man who won't drive his truck over her steep driveway and leaves her packages in the street. Then we move on to business, politics, all the rest of it. I have a feather-light awareness of her fear that if I'm not as unhappy as she is, our connection will disappear and she'll lose me. Misery not only loves company, it needs it. How are we, the few, the proud, the silent suffering, going to tough it out if everybody around us is caving to the purveyors of happy pills?

Later, when the Prozac kicked back in, I never had the guts to tell Fiona the truth. That's how we women play it, with a sort of inverse machismo. Nanny, nanny, nah, nah. I'm coping and you're not. Of course like the guy who stays up studying all night, so during the day all his classmates will think he's a genius, it's all a lie. A front, a con, an act. Our shit's all crumbling only at different rates in a headlong rush to the grave. Ahhhhhh!

The last time I saw Fiona—we live in different parts of the country now—she was taking Paxil. Apparently, she awoke in the night unable to breathe. She thought she was dying but the emergency room doctor told her she was depressed. She took exception to this diagnosis, went to a different emergency room and demanded a second opinion. It concurred with the first; and the third.

Still, the last time I was out there we went to lunch. It's what we do. You would never, say, go bowling with Fiona. I suggested we go to McDonalds. She remarked that their food's bloody awful, and was I out of my mind? I said, what's the matter Fiona, don't you like Big Macs?

She didn't get it, at all.

HMO's and Clinical Depression

I was just in the kitchen cooking eggs when the phone rang. I debated for a second whether or not to answer it because the eggs were almost done, and there's nothing I hate worse than overdone eggs. But I figured it might be somebody I like.

Wrong again. It was the behavioral health office that comes with my medical insurance. If you've been wondering what happened after Dr. Shithead, well this is it: There's a nurse practitioner that I see for ten minutes once every four months. It's my one time to touch base with my HMO provided mental health services. It was them on the phone and they said, "is this Catherine O'Sullivan?"

I said, "Yes," all the while eyeballing my eggs and wondering why I hadn't just let the machine get it. I mean, I knew it wasn't anybody important when they didn't recognize my voice.

"You have an appointment on the twenty-seventh with Ann Smith?"

"Yep," I said ready to hang up. Someone calling to confirm an appointment, I figured..., and my eggs.

"Ah," she says. "Do you need meds or anything?"

I especially like the 'or anything' part. I wanted to say yeah, you people to pay for my hundred dollar an hour shrink. But I'd tried that about five times. "No."

"Because we are going to have to reschedule the appointment."

There wasn't any smoke coming off the egg pan yet, but I knew my yolks were hardening rapidly, and these were my last two. "Ok, I said. I'm cooking my lunch right now and have to go. Just make an appointment, call me and tell me what it is." I mean, let's be realistic here. I get the chance once every four months to find out whether these pills I'm taking are making me grow a brain tumor, ruining my kidneys, heart, whatever. Chances are, I'll fit another appointment in whenever they schedule it.

"Oh, no, no, no." She said. "You'll have to do that." It wasn't necessarily what she said, it was the way she said it, like I was trying to put something over on her by asking her to rectify an inconvenience she'd caused me. Seems like *I* was supposed to rectify the inconvenience she'd caused me.

"Whatever." I hung up the phone wanting, no, needing, to hang up on her before she hung up on me.

Part of me was angry the other part felt like crying, but at least my eggs didn't burn.

So you might be saying to yourself, what's the big deal? So you had to reschedule an appointment. It wouldn't be a big deal if this was an isolated instance, but it wasn't. The truth about these people, transmitted by acts just like this played out over and over again, is that their level of concern is about equivalent to the Department of Motor Vehicles, in other words, they do not give a flying fuck one way or another.

I guess I need to backtrack.

After I stopped seeing Dr. Shithead, I got assigned to a very nice nurse practitioner. I like this kind of caregiver. The fact that their training is less than a full fledged doctor is made up for by the fact that they are interested in their work, which in this case meant me. When I met Nurse Smith, I liked her immediately. She had that intelligent, ambiguous sexuality thing going—it was obvious from her eyes, their lack of makeup, her un-dyed gray hair, her thirty pounds extra weight. Nurse Smith looked like a down-to-earth type of gal. Even her age was perfect, about ten years older than I am. There's nothing worse than having some wet-behind-the-ears kid evaluate your mental health. And Nurse Smith got it right the first time. Not only did she correctly diagnose my depression—they have to figure it out themselves even if you tell them what's wrong—she was the first person to figure out I was having anxiety problems as well. (*n.b.* Here's how most psychiatrists diagnose anxiety: They ask, "do you have palpitations and sweaty palms?" If you say yes, you have anxiety, if you say no, you don't.)

Anyway, where was I? Oh yeah, anxiety. Nurse Smith actually paid attention when I told her it felt like I had a steel belt three sizes too small, around my mid-section. She was very interested, listened to me for over an hour, made it clear that she would be available should I have any questions. She enthusiastically recommended psychotherapy in conjunction with the medication she prescribed. It's been my experience that HMO shrinks don't generally do this. They don't want people asking questions like, "If I need this, why won't my insurance provide for it?" From where they're sitting, it's better just not to bring the subject up, even if it means you're only getting half-assed treatment.

But Nurse Smith didn't seem to care. This told me I mattered more than a bunch of insurance wonks pressing buttons somewhere in Phoenix.

It took me awhile to figure out that Nurse Smith possessed her enlightened attitude for one reason and one reason only. She was new.

I'm not dissing her at all. In fact, she's a fairly enlightened individual. But if you're going to join a medical group affiliated with a so-called Health Maintenance Organization, you've either got to toady up or get fired.

After awhile I began to notice changes in Nurse Smith. The first few appointments I had weren't four months apart like they are now. They were every month, and my medications changed a few times, dosages were upped, different combinations were tried. No one thing, or combination of things, works for everybody, so getting it right is hit and miss. This is a difficult process mostly because of the way most anti-depressants work, taking between four and six weeks to take effect once you're up to the therapeutic dose. Often medications are titrated, which means you have to work the dosage up. Ten milligrams one week, twenty the next, thirty the next. You get the idea. If the therapeutic dose for a hundred forty pound woman is thirty milligrams, then you don't count the six week let's-see-if-it-works period until you're up to the full whack. Ergo, you've got three weeks titration, plus the six week it takes for the meds to actually affect your brain chemistry, we're talking nine weeks just to find out of a particular medication works. This is a long time to a seriously depressed person, but if it works, great. Everyone lives happily ever after.

But let's say it doesn't? Well, you can't just get off the shit anymore than you can just get on it. You may not have to titrate off, but you do have to let it get out of your system before another starts working. So say you're getting off something like Serzone and going on to an SSRI like Zoloft. While the Serzone and Zoloft are communing, you might feel any old thing at all, but chances are it won't be good. Maybe it will be headaches, maybe it will be nausea, maybe you will be so spaced out you won't remember your children's names, maybe you won't even remember your own. You might even come to the conclusion that it's the Zoloft that's making you sick, when of course it isn't. But how are you to know? They rarely tell you what this stuff will do when mixed with X, Y, or Z, mostly because they don't actually know. But of course they're in a much better position to make an educated guess than you are. I think they just figure it won't kill you, so they can treat you like you're an idiot if you complain. Have I mentioned I don't like psychiatrists? You call and say, "hey doc, I feel like I'm going to vomit all day." He sighs heavily and tells you everything has side effects.

It would be so helpful if they would volunteer additional

information like, it will only last a week or ten days, but they never do. I had to discover for myself that I'd get whopping headaches when starting new medication, but only for a couple of days, or maybe I'd get a buzzing in my head that made me feel like it was full of angry bees, but that it doesn't last forever either.

You're probably saying to yourself about now "well she must be a very obnoxious person, otherwise they would treat her better." Well phooey and double phooey. I am the nicest person in the world, except when I've got a word processor in front of me. I was especially nice when I was desperate and imagined the keys of the celestial kingdom resided in the hands of a gatekeeper doctor with a shitty goatee and shiny shoes.

The last time I saw my nurse practitioner, I asked her why, if I need psychotherapy, my HMO won't pay for it. She told me it's because most people stop going after three visits. I understand. The first six months I was seeing a shrink I *hated* going, and made up all kinds of excuses not to, telling myself she was no good, even though she was very good, telling myself she was just going to tell me a bunch of self-serving crap, when what I wanted was the truth, or that I was depriving my family of a nice vacation by spending too much money. Then there were the really lame excuses, like I needed to get my oil changed, take the dog to the vet to get its teeth cleaned. (I haven't had my own teeth cleaned in... ah never mind.), and the ever popular, cough, cough, I'm sick.

Oh well, of course, I said to my nurse practitioner. "Wow, aren't people lazy? They just don't want to work!" I was so self righteous and she agreed—essentially patting my hand, and telling me what a good girl I was for understanding. "oh and Catherine?" she said.

"Yes."

"Your time is up."

But that particular day as I walked out to my car, I was able to swerve and, eluding my colossal ego for just a moment, smelled a big rat. Okay, ninety percent of patients coming into Behavioral Health seeking treatment for depression quit psychotherapy after three visits. Nurse Smith's implication is that this is because by the forth visit, they start getting down to the psychological nitty-gritty, and lack the guts to get into it. Maybe this is true. I almost lack the guts to get into it and I am a reasonably gutsy person. But, let's say the average cost to see a Ph.D. psychologist around these parts is one hundred dollars an hour, which means seeing one four times a month costs four hundred dollars. In this town, four hundred dollars a month is more than many people pay for rent. Suppose the depressed person is a secretary at the local university, perhaps a single mom with a couple of kids, which is a perfectly plausible scenario. How long do you think she's going to be able to justify spending four hundred dollars a month, a considerable percentage of her take-home, maybe as high as twenty-five percent, on something like psychotherapy, even if she does need it? You average mom simply can't. In fact, I'd be inclined to guess she'd be able to keep it up for, ah, about three visits.

And even if the forgoing were not the case, (which it is) so what if Cigna, for example, has to spring for three visits. It takes a flat two hundred from the secretary's monthly pay for health insurance anyway, so the three visits will be paid for in, like, a month and a half. And of course a big HMO can whittle down a shrink's hourly fee, I would think, by as much as fifty percent. What psychologist wouldn't make a deal like that in exchange for a guaranteed supply of patients?

But okay, say I grant Nurse Smith's point and agree that the reason these people quit after three visits is simply a lack of intestinal fortitude. Let's say I grant that. They're not out that much, and maybe the secretary gets something out of those three visits. And what's the big deal about paying for the few, the brave, the ten percent who choose to stick with it? What's the big deal about paying for people like me?

Which reminds me, I've got to call Behavioral Health back today and reschedule my appointment. If there's one thing I've learned, it's that persistence is the best revenge. Those people know damn well that most mentally ill people lack the capacity, that in fact it takes everything they have just to pick up the phone and call. Shit, some of those poor stiffs are probably still on hold with that central office somewhere in northern California. With depressives or bi-polars on a downward turn, you have only to give them the old one two punch—a dismissive bovine stare combined with a gum-snapping, nail-filing dismissal and the words—the first available appointment I've got is six weeks from tomorrow, to get them to leave you alone forever.

But not me. I'm a pain in the ass, and oh-so proud of it. I can see the forest for the trees, or maybe, probably, I flatter myself. Maybe I'm just plain pissed off.

Women and a Culture of Depression

Many depressed women are depressed because of men. Not individual men, although that is common enough, but *mankind* en masse. Because no matter how we try to dress it up or civilize it, the bottom line in the evolution of virtually all mammals, is that size and strength along with the tendency for aggression, trump everything else. Women therefore, have been consigned to the number two spot in the dominance hierarchy of the meanest ape this planet has ever produced. John Lennon said it better: women are the niggers of the world.

Men may love individual women; they may crave them sexually. They may even accept them as colleagues at work but in my experience, men *do not* love women. A large percentage of them don't even like them. This is obvious enough if you look at the statistics of violence and sex crimes against the fairer sex, but it's even codified in the way we view the behavior of each. If a man has got a girlfriend in every city, if he never spends a night alone, he's a player. If a woman does the same thing, she's a slut. Women still get paid less money for equal work and possess more jobs devoid of benefits than men. We love to cast aspersions on third world countries in which the murder of female babies is comparatively common, or in which unruly wives are set on fire, but I was at the park once with my kids, and the woman on the swings next to me was busy chewing her fingernails off as she told her friend that when she had her first baby, her husband wouldn't talk to her for two weeks. He was mad at her for having a girl.

My earliest memory of the intimate touch of a man was being groped by a drunk taking me home from a babysitting job. In college I was sexually assaulted by a fifteen year old boy who pinned me against my car with his Stingray bicycle. I've been hounded to the point of mental breakdown by a swinger boss with a sock stuck down his pants, and told by another point blank that if I didn't fuck him I would never be promoted to the position I craved, no matter how good I was. When I finally gave in, he reneged on the deal. He didn't tell me I had to pretend to like it.

If these were unique experiences I wouldn't bother to mention them. But I think they are typical of a lot of women. They just don't talk about them, or more often go into immediate denial about the things that actually happen because, well, these kinds of experiences just don't jive with what we are raised to believe: that men are brave, strong, self-sacrificing and true.

But I'm not even sure these kinds of sexual intrusions and assaults do the deepest emotional damage. I think that comes from fathers who think they own their daughters, or teachers and professors who won't call on girls in class. It comes from the idea that if you haven't got a man, you are somehow less than you ought to be, or the conviction that if you're aggressive, you're a ball-busting bitch. And should you put your self interest first, the way a man does every day as a matter of course, the way he's expected to do, you are seen as deeply lacking in some essential feminine way.

The anger caused by these standards and the disjoint between the ideal and the experience is a passion that can find no path of expression. Women therefore, far more often than men, have a tendency to collapse in on themselves. We call this clinical depression.

I'm sitting in the hair salon, looking at magazines, George Clooney is on the cover, wearing a tuxedo, working those bedroom eyes. I open it up and the beautiful girls inside look about as much like the women surrounding me as Clooney looks like Keith Richards. Of course all the beauty salon women are trying like hell to look like the magazine women, but, no way. There's a lady with dyed brown hair and a bad nose job, and a tall woman with bones sticking out on her hips like a Ugandan refugee. There's a lady over there, young, great tits and the butt to match. She's not happy, I hear her say. She's thinking about liposuction for her ass, which she hates.

According to these magazines, she's supposed to have an ass like a twelve year old boy.

When I visit my mother she still sits in the same place she did when I was small, doing her makeup and hair. I remember sitting on the hall carpet, marveling at all the glop she put on her face, the ritual of it, the tools for plucking, spackling, smoothing, painting. The hair: combing, spraying, teasing, cursing roots in need of dye. And why? I could never understand why. When I'd ask her she'd say she looked like a ghost without makeup, she had no eyebrows, blah blah blah. I didn't want to have to do that when I got big. If I spent my time doing all that, there wouldn't ever be any time to play or do anything fun. Grown women had it hard. When they went to the beach they couldn't go in the water because all the glop would wash off, and they didn't wear bathing suits because they were too fat.

People asked me what I wanted to be when I grew up and I'd say a tiger. Nobody bothers tigers. I sure as hell didn't want to be a woman. It looked like a miserable ordeal. The girl next door turning into a teenager, used to walk around with her stomach sucked in. What do you do that for? I'd asked naively. She assured me when I grew up I'd have to do it to. Holy fudd, I thought. Did it never end? And shoes, guys got to wear just regular old shoes, but women? High heels. Before I even tried on a pair I'd figured out that no real woman's foot was actually going to fit comfortably into those pointy things. As far as I could tell, Chinese foot binding looked easier. Jeeze, I looked forward to wearing high heeled shoes about as much as I would eating a bowl of ground glass.

I remember a time when I wasn't judged, when it didn't matter how I looked but it didn't last very long. Those were days when boys liked you because you were as good as they were at climbing a high tree, or skating or riding a bike fast. I've always missed those long ago times of camaraderie with boys, of equality and wonder about things. My friend Jaime liked Godzilla, and I couldn't understand why, though he tried to explain it to me. He said it was because Godzilla's a fierce monster, and that day I learned that boys like fierce monsters, but I didn't particularly and that was okay.

But there came a time when it wasn't okay anymore, when the boys had to separate off and when they came back, they came back different, separate, members of a club I wasn't allowed to join. It was unspoken but nonetheless true; and as real as a brick wall.

I see women, damaged women suffering depression, anxiety, overcome by guilt whenever they enjoy their food or who can't stop eating because they can't stand the emptiness inside. I understand there's a war going on. Not something funny like Lucy and Ricky, a real war with casualties and death, ruined lives, generations of sorrow. I see women who, no matter what they do, it can never be enough. They've been struggling since the cradle and it never has been. Yet they pound away like captives against the steel reinforced walls of a prison they've colluded in the building of because of a blind acceptance of its rules.

If you think I'm just winging this shit, take a trip to Santa Monica, to the path along the cliff-side where the beautiful people jog. I've never seen so many tragedies dressed so well. Women chasing some Barbie Doll ideal that exists like one of Plato's perfect forms in the mind of Man. No one knows what it looks like, but they're all trying to be it. Lop something off my ass here, Doctor Sir. I hate my breasts; they don't look anything like Pamela Lee's. I hate my nose, and my cheek bones aren't high enough, can't you, like, put something up there, some kind of buttress and hang my flesh higher? My forehead needs another shot of botox, and my lips aren't full—the collagen's askew. My chin is weak; I always look like I'm crying, and perhaps you could prune my labia back—they don't look like the girls in Playboy Magazine. They hang down too far; I've got a bulge in my leotard. Hundred and twenty dollar Danskin and my stupid labia ruin the look.

I don't like my hair. Can you do something about my hair? It's not silky smooth but all nappy and kinked. And I'm starving to death, can you prescribe some pills for it? Look at me, I'm so fat! I counted my fat grams today and came in at a negative number. Is that possible? I mean, that should be, like good? Right? I should be losing weight. They say it's alright to use soy sauce and lemon as a salad dressing, but all that salt makes me retain water like a camel. I'm usually not this fat. It's the damn soy sauce. Maybe I'll try the unsalted. It tastes like WD40, but you have to suffer to be beautiful. Am I right?

Doctor help me please, these anti-depressants don't work. By the way, how many calories in one of these things? And listen, you're a medical man. Tell me honestly, do these pants make me look fat?

I'm not even sure happiness is possible when a person is preoccupied with the brand of nonsense this culture of appearances promotes. And who's got time to find out who they are when they're so preoccupied with what they look like? And they are preoccupied. Women who live their lives in environments like the wife and daughter of the man described earlier, the one who got mad at his wife for having a girl, have rotten self-esteem. When they look in the mirror they are *never* good enough. Feelings of worthlessness combined with the kinds of stresses and pressures life inevitably brings is a boffo recipe for lifelong sorrow.

Don't get me wrong. I like men. Hell, I have three of them (two sons and a husband) and understand fully that they too, were born into a world not of their own making. But a little empathy and a little reflection on shaking up the natural order with a view towards enlightened equality, would go a long way to finally getting all of us, instead of just half of us, out of the cave once and for all.

Epilogue: Is there a Cure for Depression?

No more than there is a cure for who you are. Most depressives hold on to an underlying philosophical conviction that life is something you struggle with and have to get through, not some wondrous blessing peopled with the likes of Santa Claus, angels, and plucky souls like Anne Frank. For us, life is a full time job administered by some cosmic administrative bureau that doesn't care whether we want to come to work or not.

But, just because you hold a conviction about something doesn't mean it's true. Philosophical convictions spring from the psychological templates. Rene Descartes wanted to prove that he existed because he didn't quite believe he did. Hegel believed history made some kind of logical sense because something at the core of his being desperately needed it to. Nietzsche placed Human Will on the ascendant because if it wasn't, he could never have survived being Nietzsche as long as he did. To say that the man was angst ridden would be like saying the San Diego freeway has a few cars.

But whereas a philosopher can argue with others until the wee hours of dawn and thereby hone his convictions to something resembling plausible, depressives live in their heads. They are forever making implausible assertions about who and what they are, then compounding the problem by selectively collecting evidence.

I don't know if low self-esteem causes depression, or if depression causes low self-esteem, but your typical depressive has a hitch in his psychological gitalong that makes him think he lacks something crucial that everybody else has. If a depressive gets flipped off on the freeway, there's a little tiny part of him who believes he deserved it. If he gets turned down for a job, a date, a promotion, virtually anything, there's a little part inside that believes whoever said no has some weird, cosmic or otherwise spooky insight into his secret and carefully guarded lack of worth as a human being.

Of course it's all false. Like the bad scientist trying to prove that all frogs are green, totally ignoring every brown, yellow, red or spotted frog he sees, the depressive's conclusions about himself and his abilities are wrong. The guy on the freeway flipped him off because he's a jerk, he didn't get the job he applied for because someone else came along who was closer to what they were looking for, the girl who turned him down for a date only ever dates men with black hair, or was simply busy that night. In short, chances are **it had nothing to do with him.** But depression's a weird kind of inverse narcissism. Everything has to have something to do with him, compelling the depressive to haul in perceived rejection and cling like a drowning man embracing a boulder.

One of the most profound *aha's* I ever had is the fact that very little has to do with me, which doesn't exempt me from moral responsibility when I'm lacking, but is just simply *true*.

The universe is billions of time bigger than my little human brain can even conceptualize. I could have a Ph.D. in theoretical physics and it would still mean that in the grand scheme of things, I know almost nothing. Billions of beings, sentient and otherwise, have come before me and will come afterwards. There are worlds in a grain of sand, legions of tragedies and triumphs going unmarked. The sun comes up every day whether I want it to or not as surely as it goes down again several hours later.

I am only as significant as I choose to be, and only in a very limited sphere. The only way I can make sense of all this is to believe that I am a small part of something bigger. Life, I guess. A multi-cellular organism that for better or for worse, inhabits this particular planet.

Tigers have claws, horses run fast. Ostriches and camels can kick like sons of bitches. Everybody has something that can help him get through. Human beings have big brains and seemingly, a unique ability to form and hold concepts. Some might argue that this is a lot more trouble than it's worth and believe me, I understand this point of view. We can create nuclear reactions but not safe ways to get rid of the waste. We invent cars but are clueless as to what to do when we're choking to death on the exhaust fumes. Psychologically speaking, we seem to have a devil of a time modifying our conceptions of reality no matter what the evidence suggests. But it is possible **and this is key**.

I am a depressive because of melancholic Irish genes combined with events that happened or didn't happen during my development. I began to crash and burn as a teenager and when I had kids of my own, suffered a complete emotional collapse. I firmly believe that had I told anyone the kinds of things I was really feeling and thinking at the time, I would have been diagnosed psychotic. I look back now and see an internal logic to it all—nothing brings you face to face with yourself like having kids—and even understand the mechanics of it, but it still scares the living piss out of me to go back there and face those times head on.

Yet in the end, I know that at the core of my problems was an extensive set of beliefs I held about the world and my place in it that were a hundred percent wrong. They were what Jung called imagos and Freud called interjects: self-destructive voices inside, programming laid down which had nothing to do with who I really was and what's more, who I needed to become. Bad software in a good machine. Sort of like Windows 98. The point is, I had to dump it, to re-program myself.

And it's not a job that's ever finished.

Survival is an interesting concept. We like to tell ourselves we're beyond the tiger in the jungle or the coyote in the desert, that we've got something wired that other animals don't have. The turd in the punchbowl however, is the seemingly unlimited capacity we have for self-destruction. What other creature literally eats itself to death the way millions of westerners are doing at this very moment, then goes home, sits in an enormous chair, and watches hours of television informing it of myriad ways to do it more effectively? What other animal routinely and constantly makes war on others of its kind? What other creature can convince itself it's okay to let its kid spend the night at Michael

Jackson's house, or that a handbag with the word "Chanel" on it is worth fifteen hundred dollars?

Being conceptual creatures is all very fine, except for the fact that most of the concepts we hold are false. I can't change the fact that politicians think it's okay to kill thousands in the name of greed and oil, nor the fact that the people who manufacture Hummers think that depicting one of these monstrosities tearing up a pristine wilderness on their commercials, is cool. What I can change are the things I believe about my place in the world and the effects my life force will or will not have. Clinical depression paralyses that ability, and what's worse, the sensitivity that many depressives possess. In other words, the very thing that made them depressives in the first place, is the very quality that could save us from warmongers and devils of whatever ilk, if only we would get off the stick and work with it.

So is there a cure for depression? No more than there is a cure for who you are. If you're down and feeling bad, maybe the treatment lies in rethinking who that person actually is.